Dancing With Belle

AF797509

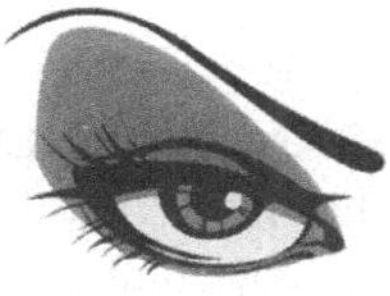

Lorraine Henegan

Dancing With Belle
Copyright @ 2021 by Lorraine Henegan
Publisher: Smiling Eyes Press

All *Rights Reserved,* including the rights of reproduction in whole or in any part in any form. No part of this book may be used or reproduced, stored or introduced into a retrieval archive, or transmitted in any manner or form (electronic, photocopying, recording or otherwise) whatsoever without written permission of the copyright owner and publisher, *Smiling Eyes Press,* except in the case of brief quotations in the context of critical reviews or articles.

The scanning, uploading and distribution of this book via the Internet or via other means without the permission of the publisher, mentioned above, is illegal. Please purchase only authorized electronic editions of this book and do not participate or encourage piracy of copyrightable materials. Your support of the author's rights is appreciated.

Disclaimer

This is a work of creative non-fiction. All of the events in this memoir are true to the best of the author's memory. Some names and identifying features have been changed to protect the identity of certain parties. The author in no way represents any company, corporation, or brand, mentioned herein. The views expressed in this memoir are solely those of the author.

Manufactured and produced in Canada
ISBN Paperback: 978-1-7771119-5-3

Editor: Dounia Royer
Proofreader: Richard Tardif
Cover Design Concept: Laurie Roche
Interior Design: Richard Tardif
Printer: Business Box, Pointe-Claire, Quebec

Dedication

Isabella Pearl Lawrence
"Belle"

Never would I have dreamed that Tuffy Belle's story would grace the pages of her own book. I thank you, Mom, for all you have been for all of the people's lives you have touched with your grace and your beautiful gift of selflessness for everyone you have loved. I thank you for all the children whose lives you have enriched with your patience and love.

And for your determined and unwavering set of standards that all children deserve to be loved and given a home together as one family, it does not mean the biggest house; home means a place to feel safe.

Preface

Belle, my mom, would often turn to me in her later years and say someone should write a book about her life. I would nod in agreement; her life had been filled with so many twists and turns, it was hard to disagree. Her stories were captivating, filled with resiliency and strength. When Covid-19 hit, and with Mom's Alzheimer's disease advancing, stealing her memories faster than anyone could have anticipated, an urgency to capture her life on paper arose in me.

When I first brought up writing this book to my family and friends, the reception I received was divided. Half said, "What a great idea! Your mom would be proud of you," and the other half gave me looks of doubt. They probably thought, "Okay, what do you know about writing?"

Well, I knew nothing. But how could I let Mom's stories disappear? I embark on penning them down. It has been an experience that I still have mixed feelings about. It has brought me to the emotional edge of my ability to stay on topic and stop crying! I thought it would be easy. Wrong. I thought it would cleanse my mind from all the pain of watching my mom slip away with Alzheimer's. Wrong. If anything, it has made me hold on to her a lot tighter.

Every chapter in the book is a story she recounted to us over the years, and once bound together, these anecdotal tales became a bird's eye view of her life. There is sadness, joy, hard choices and a lot of love. When she told her stories, she was honest, and God bless her honesty. Mom might not have always made the right choice, but she never backed down from doing what she thought was best. And she always led with her heart. I hope I have not offended anyone. I tried to stay true to the facts as I know them and the details I received from several family members.

Because of Mom's advancing Alzheimer's and the inability to question her further about her feelings during certain events, I had to jump into what I believe Mom was feeling and thinking. I do think somehow she was writing through me. I know whose daughter I am. I realize I am so much like her, and for that, I am proud.

Lorraine Lessard Henegan

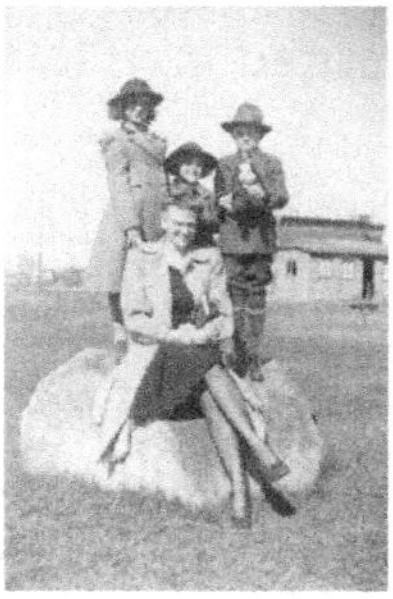

Chapter 1
Dancing With Belle

"The rule is you have to dance a little bit in the morning before you leave the house because it changes the way you walk out into the world." - Sandra Bullock.

BELLE, THAT'S WHAT THEY called me, never Bella, never Isa, just Belle. My full name on my birth certificate is Isabella Pearl Lawrence. When shortened, I am the Belle Pearl, quite poetic, but that wasn't my parents' intent.

They were naming me after my grandmother Isabella, my aunt Belle and my great-aunt Pearl. The fact that it turned out to be so fanciful is pure serendipity. I am the daughter of Zita Hertle of German descent, and Albert Douglas Lawrence of Scottish descent. My mom's Germanic features were passed down to me, a straight nose, strong eyebrows and downturned light eyes. From my dad, I took his tough demeanour and Scottish temper. I like to believe (and most say) I also inherited my mother's kindness that tempers my nature.

After my birth in 1932 in Longueuil, Quebec, my parents packed up our then family of three and moved us near Montreal's East End in Pointe-aux-Trembles, a town of farms and big oil refineries. Pointe-aux-Trembles was filled with a mix of immigrant Polish farmers, French Quebecers, and English speaking factory workers. It wasn't a pretty town to look at, with not much to offer and where the refineries smelled worse than the cattle. Eventually, though, you didn't notice the smell. That's the only place where my father could find work. My paternal grandparents urged them on as they also lived there. Dad got a job in one of the refineries. He was an operator, a position he held for 44 years. Dad worked hard; the job itself was strenuous with many long hours of hard labour with little pay.

My younger brother Douglas was born soon after we moved. And three years later, our family grew once more with the birth of my baby sister Loy. I was the oldest child out of the three and made sure everyone else knew it. I was what you call a tough, stubborn little know-it-all, ready to take on the world to protect those I loved but also to have my way.

Douglas resembled Dad in build. He had his large frame, facial features and his thick set of eyebrows. But that's where the similarities ended. Doug had a sweeter temperament than Dad. While my father's eyebrows were often furrowed in anger, which, combined with the rough tone in his voice, would make us run away, Doug was kind-hearted and patient.

Loy had long beautiful flowing black hair and was always smiling. She was such a carefree child that even Dad would soften when faced with her sweet, joyful innocence. She was the only one who was able to bend the rules without Dad punishing her.

To be fair, my brother and I also tended to push our limits and get into more mischief than Loy. And if I were frank, I'd admit Doug would often follow my lead. Dad knew this, but he still punished Doug severely. Doug began to resent him and act out by getting into fights with boys. Often there were brawls that he couldn't handle. His friends would call for me, "Belle, hurry Doug is at it again," and even though I was not the biggest compared to the boys he'd pick fights with, I would still go to help him. Doug was more than my brother; he was my best friend, and I wouldn't let anyone hurt him.

I wasn't a rebel, but I was very headstrong and loved to explore. It got me into trouble more than a few times. But even the threat of punishment wasn't enough to deter my spirit, anxious to experience life without holds or rules.

"Belle, I want you home by 8:00 PM," Dad would say, and I would answer, "For sure."

I can't remember one night that I returned on time. Dad would be mad and waiting. He'd either punish me with a smack or, if he was furious, rooster pen time.

The pen was at the farm down the road from us. Dad would walk me over to our neighbour's farm, open the gate to the pen and make me go in, and leave me in there for what felt like a lifetime. The mean rooster would spot me, run around squawking, and then he would charge me. He would peck me wherever he would reach as I stumbled around, trying to get away as I bled from my legs or arms from his pecks. Don't think I just took his abuse and didn't fight back. I would throw dirt at the rooster's eyes, and when he couldn't see, I would kick him, and it would be his turn to run away. It was like a cat and mouse game, but one he mostly won as he terrorized me in that pen and my thoughts until I got wise to his routine and would charge him before he had the chance to charge me. Dad never caught on to how I finally made that rooster afraid of me. They don't call me Tuffy Belle for nothing!

Outside of when we were being punished with the mean rooster, we loved spending our days on the farm. The farmer and his wife were sweet people; the farmer's wife would even sneak me out of the pen when my father would put me in there, and she would clean my little peck marks, give me a nice warm cup of milk and send me home. They would let us help with some of their other animals. They had some old billy goats and many large cows that we were allowed to help milk. But even when I would help with the other animals, I always felt the mean rooster kept an eye on me, just waiting for me to slip up and do something bad so he could get me back in his pen.

The farm also had a mean goat, but we never went near him; he was known as the Crazy Goat. He had crooked eyes, and I felt he could see everything from the side of his eyes; he reminded me of Dad when he was angry.

Mom, contrary to our father, was the gentler person. She had beautiful thick hair, and like Loy, she always had a smile on her face. She wouldn't go against our father or his punishments, but she made sure we felt loved by her.

Every morning, Mom would wake us a little earlier than we had to be up for school to give us the time to do our chores and to have time with her.

She would put on the radio, and we would dance and sing and dance some more. I never told anyone but these moments dancing with my mom are my happiest memories.

Later in life, my family will learn how joyful dancing makes me and wonder where it comes from, and I will not have a chance to tell them in my words as the awful disease of Alzheimer's will rob me of my thoughts.

Chapter 2
The Dancing Ends

"Mom you taught me everything I know,
But you didn't teach me how to live without you."
- Unknown.

IN 1942, THERE WERE only about six months of class time in Quebec's rural parts to allow kids to help out their parents at home. By March, school had already let out.

Our days were spent on the farm, and our nights were filled with chasing fireflies and sharing late-night secrets. I was 10, Doug 9 and Loy 5 years old. Loy would trail Doug and me wherever we went.

We didn't mind because we were more aware of the dangers around us and could protect her. Mom let us roam free to discover and run wild as long as our chores were done and that we didn't disturb our father's rest. Dad was working twelve-hour shifts.

On March 20th, all three of us kids had slept in. As we woke up, Mom was nowhere in sight to see us rushing through our morning chores.

We weren't willing to knock on our parents' bedroom door and chance waking our father, so we skipped our usual morning of dancing; instead, we decided to head outside and chase the farm cows.

Doug and I ran out the door first, with Loy following close behind, skipping and singing. What we didn't know at the time was that while we had slept the night before, Mom was sick with indescribable pain in her side.

And as we slept in that morning, Dad came home to Mom, laying in her sweat and crying out for him. "Albert, please don't let the children hear me. I need to see a doctor. Can you have one come as soon as possible?"

Within an hour, the doctor arrived and examined Mom.

He asked her some questions, and when he had finished examining her, he said, "Zita, you have appendicitis. You need to get to the hospital right away!"

"No," she said, "No hospitals, I will never go to a hospital."

"Zita," said Dad, "You have no choice. This is an emergency."

All of this happened before we woke.

As we went about our chores, wondering why she wasn't there to dance, she was dying in her room a few feet from us. We never heard her cries.

Later that day, as we came in for lunch, our grandparents were waiting for us with our father.

"I would like the three of you to sit down, please," said Dad. I knew I didn't do anything wrong. I made a mental list in my head, running through the things I had done that day, and no, I wasn't in trouble this time. All of our chores were done, we had cleaned up after our breakfast, and we hadn't gotten into trouble at the farm.

Dad looked like he was sick or had seen a ghost; he was white as a sheet. The look on his face scared me. Grandma and Grandpa had tears in their eyes, and

Grandma was visibly shaking. "Belle and Doug and you, Loy little one, I have very bad news to tell you. "

My mind raced. A hundred thoughts and questions passed by faster than it took the time to sit down. What did someone do, what could he have to tell us? Why is Grandma crying, and why does Dad seem so much scarier than when he is angry? And then one thought hit me and made me panic. Where is Mom? I need her comfort and her steadiness while all the other grown-ups are looking so serious.

"Wait a minute. Where is Mom?"

"Belle, your mother, isn't with us anymore. She died this morning." As the words were leaving his mouth, there was an echo in the room. I felt I was in a dream or that they were playing a silly mean joke. I got up and started looking around the house, "Mommy, where are you? Grandma, Grandpa, where is our mommy? Dad, where is she? We didn't make her mad or cry, we did everything she asked us to do, give her back. We didn't dance today. Is that why she's mad at us? Is she hiding, and this is all a joke? Daddy, where is she? I want my mommy. I want my mom now, please, Daddy, please!" I was sobbing as I pleaded with him. My eyes locked with my brother's, and I saw the reflection of my fear and sadness in his. I let out a hysterical scream and started to shake. Grandma grabbed me in her arms and held me until my sobs had lessened to small hiccups.

The rest of the day was a haze. I couldn't believe her hugs, and her melodious voice was no more.

Mom died an unnecessary death on March 20th, 1942, at the young age of 32.

Who was going to hold us when Dad's voice was so harsh? Who was going to make our home safe? Dad couldn't keep caring for us at the house as he worked long hours.

In the few days following my mother's death, we moved across the street into our grandparents Henry and Isabella Lawrence's home. No one asked what we wanted. It was just decided that the move was for the best. I didn't mind; I was numb with loss.

We needed stability and love to nurse us back to feeling whole. Grandma and Grandpa tried to provide that for us. We called our Grandma, Nani. She stood about five feet tall and could best be described as huggable. Nani was strict but fair. Even Grandpa, a very tall man with a deep voice, never got involved when it came to Nani making her point or her house rules. Grandpa was a big softie. He was kind, quiet and believed we were special kids. We loved to jump up on his lap and ask for ice cream, and we usually got it. Grandma would smile. She knew we had him wrapped around our fingers. But even with all their love, it couldn't take away the pain of losing Mom. I kept longing for her. I felt like we were missing the most valuable part of our family and needed her there to feel complete.

Doug, Loy and I spent most of the summer with a heavy feeling in our hearts; we were mourning without knowing how to move on from the sense of loss. Each day ran into the next and the next.

Doug, in particular, wasn't the same. He slipped further into himself every day and became more rebellious. Although we weren't living at our father's house, he would still discipline us. Everyone knew the strict rules, and that Dad ruled. Doug didn't care. He started staying out after curfew and took the spankings without flinching. Even the threat of the rooster didn't scare him anymore. The simple joys we shared before our mother's passing, be it running, playing, chasing cows, were no longer of his interest. Doug was a lost boy.

Loy was very young, which was a blessing and sheltered her spirit. The butterflies were still beautiful and worth chasing. Of course, she still missed Mom's soft embrace and soothing cooing when she woke from a fretful dream or a fall from a tree.

I tried to be there for Loy, but my heart was broken. Every time I heard her name "Zita May," or thought of her or of our moments together, the love and loss I felt caught in my chest.

Nani would come and hold us when we would wake up in the night crying for our mom. Nani was a godsend. She started healing me. We would spend quiet moments together where we would garden, and she would tell me stories of her childhood and how much she loved my mom Zita as her own daughter. As the evenings would end, I would always give her a big hug.

As the summer wore on and fall began, Nani continued to be there for me. I was diagnosed with scarlet fever. She took care of me. I was placed in a dark room for a long time. She was the only one who would risk her health for me. Nani would bathe me and bring me my food, and read to me under candlelight. The result of the scarlet fever was that I would wear very thick glasses for the rest of my life and later lose my hearing, but I would be a survivor because of her care.

Nani would do anything for us kids but could not, unfortunately, ever fill the hole our mother left.

As I got older, I wished we could have known that Mom was in distress and asked her to go to the hospital. In her fear of the hospital and her not wanting us to see her in pain, we were denied our mother. And we danced no more.

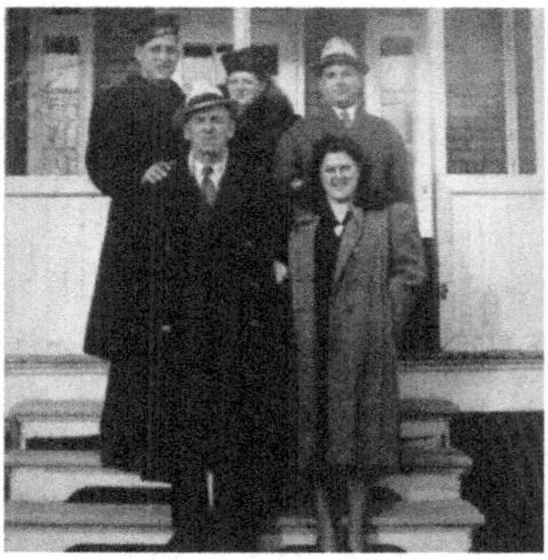

Chapter 3
Josephine

"A mother is she who can take the place of all others
but whose place no one else can take."
- Cardinal Mermillod.

WORLD WAR TWO WAS raging in the years following my mother's death. We asked Dad why he didn't go to fight since many of the other men in the town had left to serve, and he responded because he was a widower and that he had to provide for us, his three children.

He took his role as provider seriously, working many hours ensuring we didn't go without and being strict with us so we wouldn't get what he thought would be out of hand. As the years wore on, Dad felt the need to provide us with someone who could replace our mother.

He started seeing a woman named Josephine. She was heavier set than Mom had been; it was harder to picture her dancing or having the same joy of life that Mom possessed. But back then, it wasn't always about love, but sometimes about convenience.

At that time, you filled a practical need. Josephine filled that need.

They were married by 1946. It was not a large wedding, mostly family, at the minister's house, a duplex next to an old theatre on Notre Dame street in Montreal.

Four years had gone by since Mom had left us with this immense void. No one could ever replace the love of Mom, but Josephine tried to be a presence in our lives.

We still lived with our grandparents as Josephine didn't want to move us back into the house where my mother had lived and died. She urged my father to build a new home. One that wouldn't have memories. Dad said yes, wanting to please his new bride.

Josephine and Dad even moved in with us at our grandparents until the house was finished. Nani was a little thing, but boy, was she sharp. The house was hers, and Josephine stepped on Nani's toes a bit too often. Nani had her way of doing things, and Josephine refused to follow. Every night Dad would hear about it from both of them. I would listen and smile while he was stuck between his new wife and his mother.

In my mind, Nani always came out on top. Grandpa would go out back to smoke a pipe and close his ears to all of it. It was crowded and tense, but the new living arrangements had a benefit for Dad; he could keep a tighter rein on us as the months of house building passed.

Doug and I would go after school to help Dad build his new house. It wasn't going to be large, but it would serve its purpose of being a new home: three bedrooms, one bathroom, one kitchen and a small living room. After school, drop your books and pick up a hammer. We worked till sundown.

Doug was often yelled at by Dad for not keeping up with his homework, even though he had no time, as he always had to help build. The years of living apart hadn't helped their relationship.

As the house went up, and it was time to work on the roof, a fear of Doug's was brought to light, as was Dad's incredible harshness. Dad wanted him to help him put up the shingles, but Doug didn't want to climb the ladder; he was scared of heights, so Dad dropped the hammer from the roof onto Doug's head. Blood was everywhere. We stood there, mouths agape at what had just happened. Josephine brought us inside Grandma's house and cleaned up Doug's wound. Not one word was spoken about how the gash had been purposely done.

Even injured, Doug climbed the ladder the next day, still afraid of heights but more afraid of Dad.

Only Nani would have reprimanded Dad, but she was busy fighting her own battle. Nani was diagnosed with sugar diabetes. A disease that back then was seen as a death sentence.

There were no testing strips, which left the disease uncontrollable in the long term. Auntie Belle, Dad's sister, took charge of administering her needles and medications and saw that Nani was comfortable and taken care of, day in and out.

Nani fought like no other person I knew. She would never let us see her when she had a bout of weakness. Like our mother, she hid her discomfort well.

Their strength through Nani's diagnosis and treatment made me proud to be named after them. Nani endured about one year of this awful disease. She passed away as Dad's house was nearing completion.

Doug, Loy and I lost our maternal presence for the second time in our lives. When Mom died, Loy had been too little to fully grasp what had happened. This time she felt the extent of hurt and loss from death. Doug also took it hard. After Mom's death, he sought and found his soft place with Nani. Losing her destabilized him. I mourned Nani as much as I had Mom. Nani and I had a bond different from everybody else. It had been forged during my bout with scarlet fever. I knew her love knew no bounds. She had comforted me when I had lost my mother, but now there was no one to comfort me after losing her. I held my pain inside.

Soon after the funeral, we moved into the new home with Dad and Josephine. Doug wasn't happy there. He refused to accept Josephine as a replacement for our mother and rebelled at every chance.

After many run-ins with Dad, it was decided Doug would move back across the street and live with Grandpa.

I was on the fence about Josephine; I appreciated that she was trying to bring some normalcy to our lives, even though I also held it against her. Loy got along with her.

We began calling Josephine, Joe, for short. She was a house on fire; she never stopped. She took care of the home, our extended family and us three. Joe had a strict set of rules that included no dancing, laughing, and no great lemonade like our mother gave us on a hot summer day.

One time Loy and I asked if she could put the radio on for us to dance, and she said, "There will be no dancing in our house, no time, and we have jobs to do."

After a few months of living together, I was starting to see why Doug never accepted her. No matter my feelings towards Joe, I would never leave to go back to Grandpa's for the simple reason that I wouldn't want to abandon my baby sister.

At night, I would dream of Mom singing in the night breeze, and sometimes when Loy would hum with her beautiful voice, I would close my eyes and feel Mom's and Nani's love as I drifted off to sleep.

CHAPTER 4
Confession

"I say I am stronger than fear." - Malala Yousafzai.

I WILL CONFESS SOMETHING now from my childhood that was always kept quiet. I guess this was my first experience that the world has many monsters, not only in the dark or in a scary movie, sometimes they live around us in the daylight. My world of farms, dancing, and being just a kid was not to be anymore.

I don't think my brother and sister were ever told of the events I'm about to share. I know I didn't tell them, for I wanted them to keep their belief in people longer than I was allowed to keep it.

At the young age of 14, something happened to me that removed the last shreds of my innocence. I was always a lover of animals and spent most of my time at our neighbours' farm. One day, while Joe and Loy were not home, and Dad was at work, I headed to the farm to tend to the animals.

That summer had been a good one for the farm, and the farmer had hired a few extra farmhands to help. It was warm, and as usual, my first stop was to get a cold drink from the kitchen. As I turned from the barn, a hand reached out and grabbed me. In shock, at first, I thought it was one of the farmer's sons playing a prank; it wasn't, it was trouble. As I screamed for help, this hired farmhand had already ripped my blouse and was working on opening my pants, while with his other hand he fondled my breasts. I was not big. I was a skinny girl, but I was strong from fighting my brother's battles and helping on the farm. I had a chance to knee him in his ...(this action, I knew from fighting for Doug, would have my attacker hunched in pain and allow me to escape).

I ran as fast as I could to the farmhouse. By the time the news spread around the area, a group of men had gathered, led by Dad. I never found out exactly what they did to him, but I know he was taken to prison when they were finished with him. I pushed it out of my mind, not forgetting, just refusing to have it weaken me.

The years passed.

Pointe-aux-Tremble isn't a big place, and most people know one another.

That's how many years later, as an older teenager, I was quickly able to spot the farmhand who had assaulted me. He was out of place and stood out as a threat.

I was walking down the street, and as I looked ahead, I saw a very angry looking man leaning on the lamp post, and as I got closer, I could see it was him!

I screamed loud and ran as fast as I could, everyone on the street came out, and someone called the police. I don't know what happened after Dad went to the police station. I never saw the man again.

Long after, I would still remember his assault and how he tried to come after me a second time, and it would frighten me, but it also made me stronger.

I was wiser. I knew my innocence could never be recovered; it was replaced with a hardening of my resolve. A fire had been lit, and the flames burned inside me. I swore to myself that, "Never again would someone take another part of me without my consent or rob any of my loved ones, and if in my unknown future, they try, the fire inside me would surface.

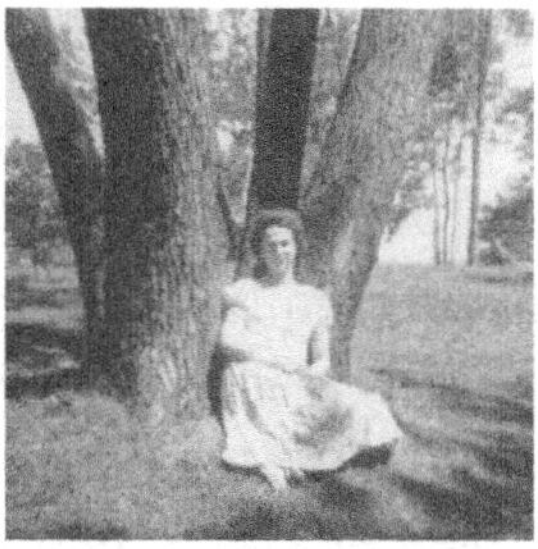

Chapter 5
Pin Curls

"I can and I will watch me." - Belle Lawrence.

IN 1951, THE WAR in Korea was getting heated, and the Allies needed troops badly. Doug saw this as his ticket to freedom away from the restraints of Dad. Although Doug wasn't living with us in the house, Dad would still discipline him, and Doug was desperate to get away.

At 17, he was too young to sign himself up to go to war. But he lied about his age and set off to Korea.

At 18, I felt my world was once again turned upside down with his departure. Before he left, I tried to change his mind. I felt I was losing not only my little brother but my best friend. "Doug, why? We have already lost Mom. I'm trying to hold on to Loy and you."

Doug just shrugged his shoulders and hugged me. That was the last hug I would get from him in more than two years. I prayed every day he would be safe.

I think even if Mom were alive, Doug would still have left. Mom did everything to make us children believe Dad loved us, but we felt that Loy, Mom, Doug, and I were the four real members of our family, and Dad was the interloper. Doug needed to leave to finally feel free from Dad.

I was the eldest, but my younger brother had become an adult before me. I still shared a room and a bed with Loy. I loved her, and we were close but, at the same time, different. Everyone loved Loy. I didn't get the same reaction. Josephine even confided in me, "Belle, you always rub your dad the wrong way."

I told her, "Joe, I am determined to be my own person," and I was. I was determined to be me. Although Josephine's comment came out of concern, it grated on me the wrong way. I wanted to explore and enjoy myself without being stifled by other people's rules and judgments. I didn't go against what they would say exactly; I just wouldn't let it prevent me from what I wanted to do. Wouldn't

I had begun going out more; neither Joe nor Dad approved. To dodge them, I would either go right after school or sneak out of the house. I would meet Marion Johnson (my best friend) and a few other girls from school, and we would go out to dances. In the winter, we would go to the rink, and I would spin my friends around the ice in a big human chain.

The faster I went, the more they would laugh and giggle.

I would come home late and have to sneak back into the house and into my bedroom. It became a routine, the same as when I would get into our bed and try and eat my chips, and Loy would ask, "Belle, can I have some?" and I would say "No." To my last day, whenever that will be, CHIPS ARE NOT TO BE SHARED, although back then I sometimes did.

It was hard to say no when Loy asked. She had Mom's sweetest singing voice, which comforted my soul. Loy also found joy in the simplest of things, and her delight in them made me appreciate them and her more. I would often end up passing her a couple of handfuls.

Even when I didn't share my chips, she would shrug it off and still kiss me good night.

Around the time of my late-night snacks was when I got into the habit of pin curling my hair before bed. In the morning, as I removed the pins, lovely soft curls would frame my face. It made me feel pretty. Pinning my hair to curl was one of my first stabs at deciding on my look and identity.

When I wasn't out with my friends, I would be out babysitting to make some pocket money. Kids loved me, and I loved them back. It felt natural to take care of them. I didn't realize at the time that working with children might be my calling in life. If I had, I might have pursued a career as a teacher.

But it was not meant to be. Not only did I not understand my career options, but I also disliked school. Education wasn't necessary or encouraged for women; society's message to young women was to stay home and have babies.

In the middle of my last year of high school, I heard they were looking for workers in a razor blade factory called Pals, so I said, "Why not?" I applied and got hired on the spot. That same day I quit school.

As I went home, I felt like shouting from the rooftops, "I have an official job!" I felt like a grown-up. I hoped that if Mom could see me, she would be proud of who I was becoming. I also hoped that Joe and Dad would begin to give me more freedom since I had done the sensible thing of gaining employment.

Dad, although happy with my job, still grumbled at every opportunity. He always found something to complain about, be it my outings or my character. At night, in bed, my thoughts would turn towards the relationship with the men in my life. It felt like I had this hole in my heart that needed to be filled. Doug hadn't returned from the war, and Dad was always working or bad-tempered. I missed the men in my family. I just wanted to be me, happy and loved. I resolved that I would find my happiness no matter what, even if it meant leaving. "Disappointment is only a time in passing; I will get to where I am going with or without my family," I would say and then would follow it with, "Why are you so hard on me, Dad? I needed you most when Mom died, and you filled yourself with other commitments. Work was your priority, and you drove my brother away with your harshness when you were present. Your strictness and duty just drove a wedge between our family. I understand you have provided for us all; the only thing we needed you to provide that you never gave, love for us all, and that didn't cost anything. God blessed you with your children. So please remember our mother and remember your gifts from God, and show us you care."

It became my prayer at night.

But some prayers go unanswered.

Chapter 6
René Oliver Lessard

"He's like a drug for you Bella." - Stephanie Meyer.

OH, HE WAS HANDSOME; he stood out with his dark hair, crisp white shirt, and black pants and shiny black shoes. As I stared quite boldly, all I could think was I am so happy I took this job. I never thought the work cafeteria is where I would find the love of my life.

I was seated in the lunchroom at work, where they served sandwiches and drinks.

And I had just spotted the most incredibly good-looking man I had ever seen and was busy gawking at his beauty.

As my eyes caught his, he smiled and walked over. "Is this seat taken?" I didn't respond because I was still staring.

Since I hadn't answered his first question, he asked me if I spoke French or English. I snapped out of my reverie and replied, "I speak both, but my mother tongue is English."

"Oh, you do talk," he said with a smirk on his beautiful face.

In Quebec, it was common back in those days to speak both languages—one at home and one outside. He told me his name was René, he spoke with a very soft voice in English. He had no French accent at all. René ordered some cokes for us in French.

Oh, he was smooth and so handsome. René was not a big man. He was quite thin and smoked cigarettes with the coolest swag. From that first day, he enchanted me.

"Do you dance Isabella, or should I call you Bella? You know, in Italian, Bella is beautiful."

"No!" I spurted out. "My name is Belle." "Same thing in French, Belle is beautiful." he said.

"Yes," I said, "I do dance. I love to dance."

We became inseparable. René and I would go dancing, skating, we would share hot chocolates at Mount Royal Chalet, we would visit friends and family, and we laughed as much as we talked. I was so enamoured by him. He was the only man I could picture spending my life with; there was no turning back now.

As we were falling madly in love, we didn't know and didn't consider that our love would cause us to have trouble with our folks.

Growing up in the '40s and '50s, French and Anglais never mixed; dating was often frowned upon by both sets of parents. I didn't care. I finally had found a love as great as my love for my mother, and soon René proposed, and wedding plans began dancing in my head. René's parents Armand and Marie Lessard were not happy about the idea of him marrying an English girl.

René's dad, Armand Lessard, was a small quiet man from the Gaspé area. Gaspé is sea and rocks with rolling hills and plenty of fish to be had. Mr. Lessard had moved to Montreal to find work outside of being a fisherman. Montreal was quite a culture shock for Mr. Lessard, as was the idea of his son dating a woman outside of French culture.

A month into our relationship, Mr. Lessard passed away suddenly before I had a chance to meet him. After his father's death, René confided in me that his dad had never really adapted to living in the city; his heart always remained in Gaspé.

René's mom, Marie Lessard, was the home's boss, and she was also the boss of René, his two brothers, Leo and Dollard, and sister Andrée. Following her husband's death, Mrs. Lessard relied heavily on her children to provide for her financially. When we met, she took an instant dislike of me. I would not let her dislike stop us, and neither would René, and luckily, the rest of his family accepted me.

Leo was the clown, and Dollard was the nicest man you could ever meet. René and I spent many weekends visiting his brothers and his friends. We always had great fun with them.

Andrée was sweet and always nice to me. Andrée never ventured far from her mom. She did have a few boyfriends, but when they would catch wind of how Mrs. Lessard never let Andrée far out of her sight, the relationship would fizzle. The extent to which her mother went to keep tabs on Andrée was daunting. Andrée had once gotten serious with a boyfriend and planned a trip to Florida. Mrs. Lessard had to go along; if not, Andrée would not be allowed. Mrs. Lessard also controlled the family's purse strings. The Lessard family was poor, which could be why her grip on finances was so firm. There were consequences to how tightly she held those strings closed, which she didn't seem to care about or notice.

René was slightly malnourished, as were his siblings. They also never went to the doctor, no matter what illness or injury they faced in childhood or as young adults. One day, while René was jumping over a steel picket fence at Mount Royal, he didn't make it over, the pike punctured into his side, and his brother Leo lifted him off. When they got home, and René was bleeding quite a lot, his mom told him, "Put pressure on it, and you'll live." Mrs. Lessard was everything my mom was not; I found her cruel and unforgiving.

My father wasn't happy about this union between René and me, either. I like to think it was because he felt he was losing another child; after one child left for war, he was now losing one to love, to René. But there were a few other reasons. My dad disapproved of René because he was French and he didn't have a job. René had quit the Pals factory and still hadn't found another position. We would be starting out with nothing, and that troubled my father.

But Josephine was ecstatic and quickly took to helping me plan the wedding. "I know it has not been easy for you, Belle, but I am going to help you with this wedding. You deserve this happiness in life," she told me.

My baby sister Loy was also happy for me; she thought René had a nice personality. Later as our engagement progressed, her opinion changed. She found he was a bit of a sweet-talker, but she gave him a chance to prove himself.

Doug was not yet back from Korea and would not be there for the wedding. I know if he were, he would have been happy for me. The wedding was planned for July 5, 1952, at the Church of Canada, Montreal East Community Church. It would go off without a hitch.

Just before the wedding was about to start, Dad asked, "Belle, do you really want to go through with this?"

"Yes, Dad, I do," and I did. Belle did what her heart said to do.

It was a beautiful wedding.

Mom's side of the family all came, René had friends and his family, and my friends were all there. My closest friend, Marion Johnston, was my maid of honour and my witness. My cousin Helene was my flower girl, and Loy was a bridesmaid. I was 19 years old, fresh-faced and filled with dreams of babies and love.

Little did I know, as I made vows to love him with all my heart forever till death do us part, became his wife and began the second part of my life, that this new life would be a bumpy ride, with many twists and turns.

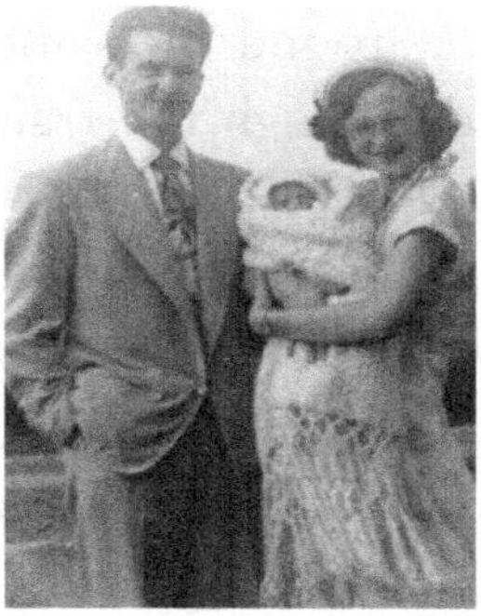

Chapter 7
Daddy's Girl

"I carried you nine months under my heart;
I carry you forever in my heart." - Unknown.

OUR HONEYMOON WAS SPENT up north with a few friends, including Andrée, her boyfriend, and Marion Johnston. We had a great time.

But we knew after this vacation, our first bump in the road had to be dealt with; we needed a place to stay. I was the only one working, and we couldn't afford to pay rent. So we moved in with Auntie Belle while René looked for work.

My René was a man with dreams in his head. Maybe because of how hard it was for him growing up, he wanted to have his aspirations come true now that he was no longer under his mother's roof.

Unfortunately, his first attempt at his dream job had fallen short. René had confided in me that he had joined the Air Force around the same time my brother had. He had passed through the training and officially graduated as an Air Force pilot. But as he was getting ready to leave for Korea, the final physical was taken, and he failed. He was given an honourable discharge. He told me how his failure devastated him; he loved airplanes and wanted so much to stay on as an Air Craftsman First Class Pilot.

He didn't confide in me the medical reason for his discharge.

His failed career made me give him some leeway as he searched to find a job that suited him. I wanted him to be happy, and luckily with my salary and us staying at Auntie's, I thought we could manage until he found something.

It took a year, and was pushed on by the fact that I got pregnant. René finally took a job at my sister's workplace. He felt valued there and seemed happy with his decision. We moved out of Auntie Belle's home and rented a small flat above a pastry shop.

Every morning we could smell the delicious scent of bread and pastries as it waffled up. It felt like comfort. With my growing belly and our home, I was content; I could picture a future filled with moments dancing with my soon-to-be child.

I gave birth to a little but perfect baby girl, May 10th, 1953, named Susan Ann Lessard. Susan was beautiful. Everyone was excited that we had our first baby. Even Mrs. Lessard was excited about our new daughter. Mrs. Lessard held her and began cooing and rocking her.

This was the first time I had ever seen Mrs. Lessard show a softer side.

René loved his little girl. He would spend many nights walking the floors to comfort her when she fussed; I thought René was the most caring and doting dad. It warmed my heart because I wasn't given the same love from my father. Dad, although he hadn't been the perfect father, was overjoyed to be a grandfather. He and Joe paid for Susan's baptism and the celebratory dinner afterwards.

After Susan's birth, when the newness and the excitement started to die down, a new dream and passion popped up into René's head. He wanted to become a famous photographer. He started to spend a big part of his paychecks to make this dream come true. He'd even spend part of our rent money on development materials for the pictures. I would try and get him to realize we couldn't afford such an endeavour; it didn't suit a young family with barely two pennies to rub together. René would sulk and leave for a few hours and come home feeling sorry.

I would fall for it every time. Have you ever heard the song by Billie Holiday, "When a Woman Loves a Man?" I felt the lyrics, "When a woman love a man...She'll be the first one to praise him...When he's goin' strong...The last one to blame him...When every thing's wrong," was how I wanted to be with René. I wanted to reason with him, but in no way blame him or dash his hopes.

Things got worse. He quit his job at the company. I didn't understand why he would leave and spoke to Loy.

She said he was well-liked, and everyone was surprised he resigned, even the boss.

My family and friends helped us financially when they could, but times were tough for everyone, and we couldn't rely on their assistance. It wouldn't be enough to sustain us. René got another job but didn't keep it for very long. It was the beginning of a lifelong pattern. Every time he liked a job, and everything was going well, he would quit, back to the photography dream. Money became our biggest problem. I would go to the food bank and the Salvation Army to pick up baby clothes for Susan and occasional furniture. Even with my frugal spending, we couldn't afford the apartment any longer and moved out and into a rooming house.

We slept and mostly lived in our room. There was a communal stove and bathroom in the hallway. I would wash my little Susan in the sink of the shared bathroom. I would try to clean the sink with soap beforehand. Susan was the cutest toddler; she was so tiny yet determined to walk at a young age, but I didn't feel safe with her crawling and exploring in the rooming house. The halls were never swept, and it stunk of sewage, and you had to hold your breath while walking in the halls. Another concern was the rats that ran rampant all over the property. The rooming house was next to a meat market, which drew in rodents. I would spend the next part of my life chasing away rats. The stench of the rats sticks to your nose hairs. It's like the smell of death and disease. I had never encountered a rat before; even on the farm, the cats took care of them. I was not raised in a fancy house, nor was I a rich girl, but I had been fortunate to live in a warm and clean house that had been rodent-free.

My first encounter with a city rat was quite the episode. I was walking down the hall from the common bathroom, and I heard a noise. I looked around to make sure it wasn't a transient. Oh no, it wasn't, it was a rat the size of Nani's cat. My first instinct was to run and not look back. However, being Tuffy Belle, I decided I would take it on. How foolish I was. I threw my hairbrush at it and missed. It started to advance, and what did I do? I ran as fast as I could into the room and slammed our room door where René was rocking Susan to sleep. His eyes popped out, "What is wrong, Belle? Be quiet. Susan is almost asleep."

The next day I found a big piece of wood lying outside and brought it in as my weapon. I vowed, "I have conquered a mean rooster, at least 20 big boys, and a sexual deviant; there's no way I am going to run away from a small dirty mammal again. My baby lives here, oh no, I'll get them they will not pass this door." But they wouldn't pass by the door but by the vents. True to my word, late at night, I would beat the life out of any rat that entered. I would wake with their smell, flick the lights and batter up, I'd club them. I said a long time ago the fire in me is there, don't wake it.

Chapter 8
The Trunk On Wheels

"Do not pray for an easy life, pray for the strength to endure a difficult one." - Unknown.

I NEVER THOUGHT I would end up like this. The refrain, "Belle, we can't pay the rent this month. We are going to have to leave tonight," became a constant in my life, and I would respond, "Alright, I will go and pack up my trunk."

The trunk and our meagre belongings in it were all we had. I don't remember when it was, but at some point, someone had given me a trunk on wheels, and it became my treasure chest. I would drag it everywhere we would live. If we were evicted, all of our worldly possessions would be in there.

I would wrap Susan in blankets, pack the few clothes we had, and at night we would leave to avoid having to pay. I would put my pride aside and go to the church and beg for milk or food for Susan to eat, while I would go without.

I would knock on many hostel doors, saying I would do chores, cleaning, cooking anything if they would offer to let us stay.

Before our second year of marriage was up, we had already moved countless times. René was jobless again, I was pregnant again, and we were homeless, again. We found a shelter, but it was only for women and children. René couldn't come with us.

"Belle, you stay here, and I will go to my mom's, and as soon as I get some work, I will come back for you." His mother wouldn't accept me to stay in her house. I agreed to go to the shelter.

The women's shelter could only house Susan and me for a short time. I was helping out to compensate for the cost of my food and lodging. But even with the help I provided, I knew I couldn't stay too long. It felt like an eternity before René came back. But it was my anxiety that made it feel so long; he was back as promised in as little as a week. He had found a job in Richelieu at the Bennet shipping factory.

It was a long train ride to work for him, but it allowed us to move into a new rooming house. I continued to pick up food at food banks and all Susan's clothing at used good stores. Unfortunately, another thing was a mainstay; rats, rats, rats. Over the last few months and rooming houses, I learned to block the vents of the rooms with steel wool and broken glass, to keep out the rodents. I would never be afraid of them again. I refused to break down; no matter what confronted us, I found a way to make due.

Precisely 11 months after Susan's birth, our first son was born, Daniel René Lessard, April 1st, 1954, April fool's day. Mrs. Lessard was ecstatic, a boy, she was so pleased he would carry on the name Lessard. Our families were all happy for us and gathered to celebrate our new addition.

Auntie Belle showered us with hugs and small presents. My uncle Bob, who had recently returned from Germany, came with his gorgeous gypsy wife, Sonya, who had bought adorable knitted clothes for Daniel. René's' brothers, both recently married, Leo to a sweet woman named Louise and Dollard to a beautiful English woman named Gertrude, also brought gifts for the first boy to be born in between them. It seemed like a picturesque celebration and show of support for our young family, but there was one thing errantly pushed to the side. Almost no one acknowledged or wanted to bring up the truth of our situation; we were poor and suffering and had no way of providing for our growing family.

Maybe they believed it would go away if they didn't talk about it. That was also true for me. I refused to recognize how bad our circumstances had gotten.

The only one who showed concern was Dad. We went to visit him and Joe at their house. Dad loved his new grandchild, but the poverty we lived in was a worry for him.

Although he was a gruff man, he wanted his children to be happy in life. "Dad, I am happy I live with the love of my life, and I have two beautiful children that I adore. Happiness does not always come easy, but if you measure it by love, I am the happiest woman in the world."

Our beautiful Susan was not happy with her new brother. At almost a year old, she was daddy's little girl and was used to being the center of our world; you could practically hear her thoughts as she made faces at her new sibling. "Who is this kid taking all the attention from my mommy and daddy." Susan didn't like it or him.

As the months passed, I noticed that my Irish twins got along like oil and vinegar; they didn't mix well. René adored them both and spent many hours with them. He loved his children and didn't notice the jealousy brewing between them.

By the time Susan was two, my quick little girl let me know she was not impressed with her brother and showed me that I would need to keep my eyes open around them.

We were in our room at yet another boarding house, and Susan was by her brother's bassinet. When I went to the other side of the room, Susan took a blanket and covered her baby brother's face.

I was looking for some clothes for the baby, and I looked up and saw her. I thought Susan was maybe playing peek-a-boo, but as she swiftly pressed down, I couldn't rationalize it.

I yelled, "Susan! What are you doing?" I rushed to the bassinet and removed the blanket, and Susan started to cry.

I never told René; he probably would not have believed it anyway. I also never spoke to her about it, but she talked about it as the years passed and found it quite funny without a stitch of guilt. This is why I said oil and vinegar don't mix; I prayed as a mom that one day they would get along.

I loved my children so much my whole universe was focused around them. I would do anything to make sure we stayed together, and they had what they needed. I hadn't held a regular job since I had Susan, but I was always trying to make a little money to keep us afloat while not taking away my time with them. When René would go to work, I would take in other children to babysit. It wasn't a lot, but I just loved kids, and the extra money helped out.

Even with the extra I would make, it wasn't enough to keep us housed as René would either squander his pay or quit another job. Evictions were a constant, as were the rats and cockroaches.

I would bundle up the kids, carry all I could, pulling my trunk on wheels, and find a shelter willing to take us. Why couldn't René keep a job? Why did he always put me in a position where I would have to plead for assistance? "Please Reverend, can you spare a loaf of bread? Or can we sleep here?"

Mrs. Lessard would always welcome René into her home while the kids and I had to fend for ourselves. René would say, "Belle, I promise I will come back for you and the children."

My days would then be spent going to different government offices asking for help, and they would tell me to separate from René, and then I could get more money. "Never would I leave my husband." I'd respond and march out of the office. I would bundle up Susan and Daniel, put them both in the carriage and walk to food banks pulling my trunk behind me.

Many days, we went without or close to; I was malnourished, and the kids were always hungry. Everything I'd be able to get went to the children. Later on, I would realize that love is blind. René had no problem quitting work and leaving us to go to shelters while he was at Mrs. Lessard's place fed and warm. I was in love; I would do anything for love. My children were my world, but my husband held my heart.

A few times, Mrs. Lessard would let us all come over for supper, but she was still as cold as ice.

René's sister and his brothers would pass me a little money without René seeing, and Andrée would tell me, "Belle get some food for you to eat; you are too thin." I never did; it was tucked away for food for the children. How could I spend it on myself?

When we would go and visit Dad, he would do the same thing. I felt so much shame facing Dad. I wanted to prove to him that we were alright but at the same time, I was starting to feel like the only good thing I ever accomplished in my life was my children, who were suffering greatly. I had so wished to be able to be the mom my mother had been, to dance with them, to cook for them, but instead, I could only concentrate on survival and if we'd have somewhere to lay our heads the next night.

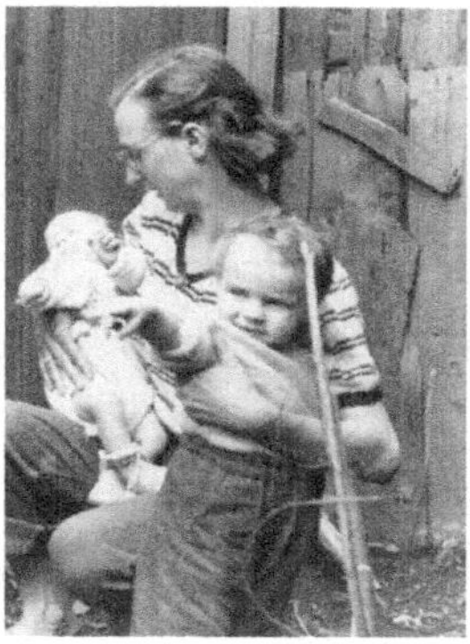

Chapter 9

The Dangers Of Rooming Houses

"Let me not pray to be sheltered from dangers, but to be fearless in facing them. Let me not beg for the stilling of my pain, but for the heart to conquer it."
- Rabindranath Tagore.

OUR LIVES HAD FOUND a bit of a routine as I tended to the kids and tried to keep us in clean clothes and our room tidy, while René was out and about either at work or his mother's.

Growing up, I had been taught to keep my person neat and the house spotless. Even though the rooming houses were not clean, I would insist René buy Javel bleach so that our room could be.

Javel was essential no matter where I lived or how much money we had because even if it was home for just a short while, it had to be clean. The same went for the kids. I would scrub their clothes in the tub and wash them with soap in the sink.

As Susan started her terrible twos and Daniel had just turned one, I became pregnant with our third child. I began going to bed at the same hours as the kids, not waiting for René to come home.

One night, while I was deep asleep and René was at work, a man broke into our room. I woke to the sound of Susan fussing.

Daniel was sleeping in his bassinet, and Susan was next to me on the mattress. I don't know why I never heard him come into the room.

As my eyes adjusted to the darkness, I saw him, short and burly looking, hunched over our bed. A flash of white fury hit me; this man was undressing my Susan. Susan was two!!! Criss de Cochon!!!

I reached down by the side of the bed, where I kept my rat bat, and I struck him. I think I cracked his skull. He started stumbling.

I jumped up, bat in hand and kept on him as he tried to escape by the door. I pushed him so hard backwards that he fell down the stairs outside of our room. I locked the door, turned on the light, and tried to comfort Susan back to sleep.

I couldn't understand how he got in; I was sure I had bolted the door that evening. My only guess was that in my haste to put the kids to sleep, I hadn't turned the lock fully.

René got home a little later than usual; maybe he had stopped by his mom's house for something hot to eat. I never thought to ask.

I jumped up fast to open the door. I flew into his arms, crying. He looked stunned, "Belle, what has happened? Are the kids okay?"

I blurted it all; the words were spewing out of my mouth. Daniel and Susan started to fuss, so we stepped into the hall. "Belle, tomorrow we will go with my brother Leo in his car to the countryside. I will show you how to shoot a handgun." His mouth had thinned into a determined line, the danger our daughter had been in affecting him.

"René, I would feel so much safer." That night he held Susan and me tight.

Bright and early, Leo came to pick us up. Leo said he was hungry and had not eaten yet, so he offered to bring us to a diner for some hot breakfast. It was a diner that he, René and their father had often stopped by before going to the countryside to hunt. They used to love going hunting together. When we first started dating, René had even brought me in front of his parents' house to show me the deer he had shot; it was tied to the trunk of his old Vanguard, a big car that was just slightly smaller than a pickup. They had not often made the trek up north since their father's passing and never with the kids.

Susan was thrilled; Daniel was happy to sit in the highchair, sucking on toast. We didn't do outings like this often; restaurants and long car rides were all new to them. Leo was laughing, enjoying the time with the kids. He loved children.

After breakfast, we set out for the hour drive north to the Laurentians. We got to a big field where Leo parked the car, and he and the kids stayed in the vehicle. René and I got out, and he showed me how to unlock and load the firearm. As I practiced, he set up a target for me to hit. I must have been a sharpshooter in another life. The gun, a 45 Colt pistol, fitted my hand perfectly, and even though I wore such thick glasses, my aim didn't take long to perfect. René was an avid hunter, a good shooter in his own right, and I sure impressed him that day. Although, I think he was also a little worried about how firing the gun thrilled me. I would cheer every time I hit the target.

The children were happy with the adventure, Leo, in helping us out, René in the knowledge that his wife could handle herself, and I was delighted with my new skill and weapon. The gun was mine to keep, and it would be well hidden, hopefully never to be used outside of target practice. We returned to the city, everyone smiling.

Chapter 10
Sweet Song Bring Me Back

"You may not control all the events that happen to you, but you can decide not to be reduced by them."
- Maya Angelou.

OUR DAUGHTER CAROL WAS born on October 30, 1955. René was suspicious of Carol; he began to say she was not his and accused me of having an affair with the milkman. This was so ridiculous. I spent all of my days at agencies begging for help; we could not afford milk!

Nothing seemed to dissuade him from thinking I had stepped out on our marriage. The more I protested my innocence, the more he steadfastly denied that Carol was his daughter. I was at a loss as to how to get through to him. Later on, I would realize that guilty people accuse the innocent as a way of masking their secrets. I was so upset and hurt by his insinuations; I stopped speaking to him for days. Unable to believe that he thought so little of me or the commitment we had made to each other.

He used Carol's physical appearance as ammunition against me. She didn't look like our other children. Susan and Daniel both resembled their father.

Carol was more like me in looks, but her hair was beautiful and thick. Carol's hair was just like my sister Loy's. I wished he could see her for who she was, our beautiful daughter. He left for his mother's house and then came back a week later. The tension was high, but we didn't argue about it anymore.

As the months passed, we eased back into how things were before he accused me of cheating. Money was tight, and neither of us could afford fighting or to hold grudges or hurt against one another. We, for better or for worse, we're a team. René would watch the kids when he wasn't working, and I would go clean other people's houses or babysit here and there. I still hoped we could have a happy-forever home someday.

When I had free time, I would take the kids out to the park, and they would run and laugh and play. When the three of them were together, I would remember us three Doug, Loy, Belle.

Running like the wind could not touch us, the feel of the sunshine on our skin and the sweet smell of summer grass. I often thought of those days, and I questioned, why did I run? Why did I not soak those moments in with my siblings to make them last forever? As adults, we still loved one another, but the closeness and the carefree spirit we all had was no longer. I missed it.

When Doug returned from Korea at the end of the war, he brought back a few ghosts with him. War changes men. It changed Doug; he became more withdrawn. I never asked Doug what happened over there. I didn't want to ask him questions about a time he would rather forget.

Upon his return, he was trying to find his footing; jobs were scarce. Doug was stubborn and hardworking; he wouldn't stop searching and was ready to accept any position available. He took a job shovelling snow. When spring arrived, he found a job on the new canal in Montreal, blasting stones. Work and his new sweetheart Lise, a friend of Loy's, kept him busy. I was busy with my babies. We didn't spend much time together. Doug was determined to succeed in his life, maybe to prove it to Dad or perhaps to prove it to himself.

By 1955, he was sent to work on a canal in Ontario. He took Lise along. That Christmas, they hosted a Christmas party in their apartment over there. They surprised their guests by turning it into a wedding. He got married, surrounded by his new friends, all for the low cost of $10. I was not there, nor was Loy or any other family member. He hadn't confided in his wedding plans. And even if he had, Carol was only a few months old, and we hadn't the money to go to Ontario.

Doug and his new bride returned to Montreal shortly after with plans of starting their family. A new strain on our relationship popped up. Lise and I rubbed each other the wrong way; she was so bossy with my brother. I guess I never stopped being his big sister and wanting to protect him from those I felt bullied him.

We would occasionally get together in the park in the summer, or go skating on Mount Royal in the winter. It wasn't often, partly because of our schedules but also because of my pride.

I felt they looked down on me and my family's poverty and worse that they felt bad for us. I could feel it every time they would come close to kiss me on my cheek. They wouldn't look into my eyes as they came near. It's like Doug didn't want to see what was really happening to me. Maybe because then he would have felt obliged to have words with René. I can't blame him, for I also vehemently swore I was fine. He listened to my words, and I think he was embarrassed to investigate any deeper, and to ask questions that couldn't be taken back or avoided. Those moments made me keep to myself more.

Every visit with Doug and Lise, even if they tried to pretend that all was normal, they would do something that most adult siblings won't do, they would push money into my hand. Lise always insisted. She loved my kids and would nudge Doug to give me money. She would tell me, "For the children."

My relationship with my little Loy also had changed over the years. She was now a busy young woman. Almost 20, she was always working and was preparing to settle down with her beau Russell. Russell was in the army. They had decided to tie the knot later that year in Nova Scotia since he would be transferred to a military base out there. It would mean we'd be unable to attend her wedding and this saddened me greatly. As the date of her departure approached, I tried to visit her more. I'd go by her place, or on weekends we would also catch up in the parks while the children played.

I never wanted my family to see where we lived and how we lived. I am the oldest but not the wisest; it seems. I did not want them to look down on us. I was proud, dirt poor, and they knew, but I tried to shield them from seeing us that way.

Loy, just like Doug, would slip some money in my hand. It broke my heart each time. "Belle, you have to stop begging, you have to make him work," she'd say. "René has to keep a job, and you have to stop having kids. I fear for you, Belle, I fear for you."

As always, I would say, "Loy, I am a big girl. I know what I am doing. I will pay you back one day. You can sing me a sweet song as you did in our rooms and make me smile again, just one sweet song, to bring me back."

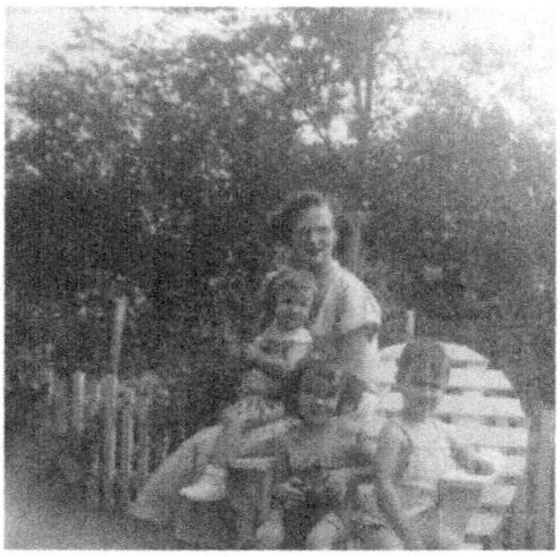

Chapter 11
No One Should Ever Go Hungry

"She will not go hidden for her strength
will not allow it." - D. Henegan.

WE MOVED INTO A rat-infested flat in the basement of an apartment complex in the sector of Westmount, Montreal. Outside, smelly homeless bums were always begging on the street.

The flat was humid, and again I used Javel, hoping to bleach it clean for my young family.

This dirty apartment did have one thing going for it; two rooms, which with our kids getting older, we desperately needed. Susan, our mini-boss, was five, Daniel, a loud four, and our youngest, Carol, two years old. Susan and Daniel would fight over everything.

Complicating things even more, Daniel was not impressed with Carol; he wanted a brother, and from the start, he had it in for her. I often had to keep them separate; during those times, the multiple rooms were a blessing.

I was pregnant with my fourth child, and I would hear comments from friends and family when they thought I was out of earshot, "When is she going to stop having babies? Does she realize she is poor and can't afford them?"

I heard it all, and yes, some of it stung when it came from the people I loved. On the darker days, I asked myself the same question, Why did I keep having children? None of my answers seemed like the right one. My Frenchman did love making babies, and I might have taken his lovemaking as proof of his love.

Or was it a way for me to give the love I lost from my mom's death? Or was it that even though it would take a toll on our well-being and finances, I saw a baby as a miracle, and when it happened, I made room in my heart and home. When I told René I was expecting again; I tried to bargain with him, "One more mouth to feed; I will just eat less." René didn't respond.

Daniel was excited because maybe I would finally bring home a boy. Susan, my mini-boss, was already helping me with the chores. She would watch Carol and sometimes Daniel, while I would take a short nap. I was often tired.

I was malnourished during this pregnancy, and the lack of nourishment showed. I couldn't think about that. I was ready to give birth.

I left the kids at home; I was told a nurse would come tend to them during my stay in the hospital.

Jo-Ann Isabelle Lessard was born December 8, 1957, a beautiful dark haired baby with jet black eyes and curly long black lashes. Jo-Ann was always crying. I commented on it, but the hospital staff said nothing was wrong, probably just gas. I knew from my other kids this baby had a problem; she cried way too much for it to be gas. But with the doctors telling me it was nothing, there was not much for me to do but return home.

Daniel was quite anxious to see the new baby. As we arrived, little Daniel pulled back the blanket and gasped, "Not again! Mommy, you said I could have a brother!"

Susan and Carol were thrilled. Susan was already talking about dressing Jo-Ann up in pretty little dresses. They were fascinated by her pretty lashes and dark eyes because they had blue eyes.

The day after I brought Jo-Ann home, Carol was sick. She wouldn't eat, had a fever that wouldn't go down and chills. I was frantic; I took her up to the Montreal Children's Hospital. She was diagnosed with tuberculosis. I found out the nurse sent to our house had tuberculosis and had most likely infected Carol. Jo-Ann, my newborn, was immediately taken up to the hospital to be tested for the disease; she was given some antiviral medications to make sure she had a chance and thank God she was okay.

After three trips to the Children's Hospital, the situation was bleak; Carol was taken to the center for infectious disease located on Nuns Island and put in incubation. The doctors warned me it might take months or years for her to recover, that is, if she ever did. If you have had a sick child, you would know how those words from the doctor tore my heart. I felt overwhelmed with guilt. I thought it was our fault she caught this terrible virus. If we had been living in better circumstances, maybe she wouldn't have gotten sick.

René was always working or not at home. I would go up to the center by myself. Unfortunately, I didn't go as often as I should because getting to the center was not easy. It required money and time, two things I didn't have much of; cash for bus fare and time since I had a newborn at home.

René would not give me his full pay, and most of the money he would give only covered the rent and food for the kids. When I could save up enough bus fare, I would leave Susan, Daniel and baby Jo-Ann with a friend, Mrs. Craig. I would take the 30-minute bus ride to Nuns Island and visit my Carol.

René had introduced me to Mr. and Mrs. Craig, but he never told me how they met. René had lived up to my sister's thoughts of him being a sweet talker; he was a charmer, and he knew how to say just enough to explain a story but keep parts of it hidden, to conceal his whereabouts and motives. René asked Mrs. Craig to keep an eye on me with the children, pop in, and spy and make sure we were all right. She was very friendly to me, and I appreciated her help and company. I had no idea about this arrangement she had with René to spy on me until later. And when I found out, my only thought was if René was so concerned, he should have helped out more or been home.

Mrs. Craig would watch the children and feed them what she could. This help was essential for me; I was close to being a broken mother. Carol was kept in the ICU on Nuns Island. My daughter was living in a plastic tent, and I was of no help to her. René never went up to see Carol. I asked him why. René wouldn't give me an answer. I wouldn't talk to him again for a few weeks in disgust over his rejection of our child. It seems I was the sole parent of this beautiful daughter of mine.

Doug and Lise would go up when they could, and I would be forever grateful for this. Loy, who had moved back from Nova Scotia, would also go and sing to her, and she would fall asleep.

René and I were going through a difficult time. We were evicted once again. René went back to his mother's house, and I had to go back to a shelter with my kids and my trunk, unable to see Carol during this time. My mind was so overcome with my uselessness with my daughter that it rendered me numb; I couldn't process it. The only reconciliation was that I knew she was receiving the care that I couldn't provide. My hands were full trying to keep my other kids fed and safe. It was the only thing I could do.

I would ask my mini-boss to watch baby Jo-Ann at the shelter so that I could do the laundry or chores. That's when I saw her do something that hurt my heart and question what I had done to my children. Susan was so hungry she stole her baby sister's milk bottle and drank it. Susan was starving; I couldn't blame her. I never said a thing to her, my poor first baby.

Little by little, my world had become not what I thought it would be, but I had my babies, and I loved them, and I would do anything to keep us together.

René came to get me, he had found us a rooming house to stay in, and he had landed a new job. I left with him and brought my kids and my trunk, hopeful once again that it would be better this time and we'd have seen the last of shelters and hunger.

Chapter 12
Make A Wish

"Let them eat cake." - Marie Antoinette.

THERE'S ALWAYS A HONEYMOON period when René and I get another place to stay. A period of renewed hope and affection. That honeymoon period often resulted in a pregnancy. That was the case in 1959, I was expecting our fifth child, and René was holding down a full-time job. It appeared we were slowly figuring things out.

It had been almost two years since Carol had been taken to the center. She seemed to be healing from tuberculosis, and the world felt just a little brighter because of it. But I had lost out on bonding with her during those years. It was hard. I couldn't visit often, and when I would visit her, we spoke in French as that was what she now had gotten used to; all the nurses at the center were French.

As my due date approached, I went less to see her but was comforted that hopefully soon she would be back home.

Labour started early on the morning of April 1, 1959, while René was at work. Alone, I walked from the rooming house to the hospital.

By the afternoon, my newborn was in my arms. René Robert Lessard was born with dark sea blue eyes and dark curly hair. Baby René's eyes were as big as buttons, and he did not cry much.

As he would get older and cry at everything, we would call him René Baby-La-La.

A few days later, when I arrived back home, I called Daniel over and said, "Daniel, come and move back the blanket, please."

Daniel looked at me and said, "Mommy, I don't want you always to bring a girl."

"Come close to Mommy, Daniel, and look at your new brother René. He was born on the same day as you. I know God had a plan for you both to forever share your birthdays together." Daniel had the biggest smile on his face as he touched René and said, "I am your big brother! Thank you, Mommy!"

The year 1959 continued on a higher note than the years that had passed before.

Carol would be returning home right before her birthday. I was incredibly happy even though her return wouldn't be the smoothest. She had a hard time speaking English because of the constant exposure to French at the center. We would have to teach her the English language all over again. Carol had developed a speech impediment and would have to receive speech therapy. Carol also lost one lung's full function due to this disease and would spend her life fighting many bouts of croup cough and pneumonia.

I felt wracked with guilt over her rough start in this world; a father who rejected her, the two years spent with strangers, and her ongoing health problems. But I was also happy to have her home.

We had never really celebrated the kids' birthdays. As Carol's fourth birthday was coming up, I wanted to change that. I stashed enough money to spend on a cake for her. I packed the younger two kids in the carriage and told the older ones to get ready.

It was late October, and there was quite a chill in the air. Luckily Auntie Sonya always made sure my kids had warm mittens, hats, and socks. She was kind to my children and tried to provide them with things that would make them smile. Sonya had been a gypsy dancer in Germany. She was lighthearted and had a giving spirit that even the atrocities of war could not squash. Now that she was married to Uncle Bob, Sonya had stopped dancing but still tried to give others joy, even if it was in the form of crazy coloured warm socks.

The kids dressed warmly in their colourful apparel, and we headed up to Steinberg's grocery store. The children helped me pick out the cake. They chose a chocolate cake, two round layers with dollops of chocolate icing. They giggled and smiled as the cashier wrung it up.

After supper, I brought it out. Carol's eyes lit up with joy, and the other children were thrilled about this rare treat.

René had gone to his mother's for supper. He walked in at that moment, "Belle, where did you get the money for that cake!"

"René, I put it aside and spent less on bread because I would skip my portion."

"How could you!" he yelled. "You wasted money on her, and she isn't even mine." The kids started to cry. I turned to Carol and saw the look on her face. She knew what he was saying.

I felt ashamed for letting this man hurt her this way. René stomped out and went out to his mom's or brothers'. I gathered up the children and plopped Carol on my lap, and we all sang Happy Birthday, the best we could. I held her a little tighter that night, and I hummed a tune I learned from my mom when I rocked her to sleep.

This outburst of René's wasn't typical of how he was with our children. If I had to compliment René, it would be that he was always gentle with them, he hardly ever raised his voice, and when he was home, he took them out to the parks or to visit his brothers. Although he wasn't affectionate with Carol, he didn't let Daniel or anyone else get away with hurting her. Daniel didn't like or treat Carol well. Once, while I was busy with the younger children, he tried to hang Carol inside the cupboard. Susan came to get me. René spanked him hard for that, and it wouldn't be the last time that René took him over his knee because of his actions against his younger sister. Daniel received many broken bats on his butt to leave her alone.

The birthday cake had been my way of giving the children a small taste of pleasure and fun, as I had so often had with my mother, Nani, and at our neighbours' farm. I wanted the children to experience contentment and full bellies.

What I wouldn't have given for them to know the smell of fresh eggs cooking, bacon in the pan, and the sweet taste of milk fresh from the cow. I wished they could run with the cows and goats and laugh till their faces hurt. The life we were leading was not the one I would have chosen, but it was the one my children would have to bear.

They were surviving off of powdered milk (when we could afford it) or water instead of milk. If there was any extra formula for the baby, the other kids would have that instead of water. Our main staple was usually bread mixed with sugar and water. I never ate until there was sure to be enough for my children. The small celebration for Carol was another slash in my relationship with René. We seemed to be moving further and further apart. I tried to find ways to hold us together.

René had switched to working nights driving a taxicab, and he always wanted his shirts crisp and white. It meant extra washing for me, but I hoped he would see I was trying to be a good wife. Laundry was a chore. We could never afford a washing machine living in a rooming house, so I would drag out the washboard and scrub all our laundry, including the cloth diapers. Ugh.

Since he wasn't there in the evening anymore, I made arrangements to earn some extra money by watching the floors at night in the rooming house. The rooming house consisted of three floors. My job was to make sure no transients or drunks were in the halls. I'd have to kick out the drunks at night, and when they would give me a hard time, I would punch them in the face. They didn't see it coming and would never come back. Tuffy Belle was on the job. If only I could have gotten through to René as I did with everyone else.

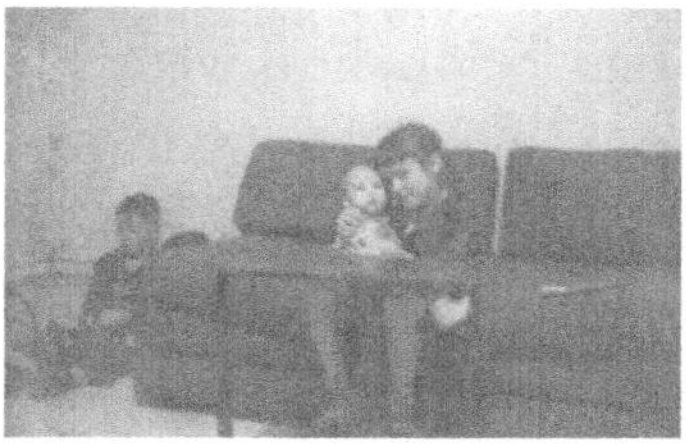

Chapter 13
The Baby

"For the youngest child,
the rules don't apply." - Lorraine Henegan.

AT THE AGE OF 32, I now had five kids and one on the way. "Isabella je ne peux pas croire que tu es à nouveau enceinte? L'enfant ne peut pas être de moi!"

"René, how can you say the baby is not yours? I have known only one man, and that is you."

There was no reason to doubt the paternity of any of our children. I had no spare time to even contemplate cheating on René! Having been through this song and dance with him before, we argued, but I wasn't as hurt as I had been the first time when Carol was born. It seemed like a tactic to give him an excuse to stay at his mother's more often. I didn't understand why he wouldn't allow himself to be happy with us and felt the need to leave our home.

He had reasons to stay, a wife who loved him through thick and thin, sons and daughters who looked up to him. And for the first time out of all the years together, René had a job he loved. He had landed a prestigious position as a chauffeur for the head of a wealthy Montreal family (for discretion, I will call him Mr. B). He was surrounded by the upper class. He wore freshly starched white shirts, a black suit, and shiny black shoes. René loved to be well dressed and be around wealth.

When he would be all dressed up for work, it reminded me of the first time I met him. He looked handsome and smooth. The only negative part of the job was that he was required to work long hours and be available at all times. However, that didn't seem to bother him much.

The first year of René working for them was also the first year we had plenty of food at home. This sixth pregnancy would be easier for me since, for once, I wouldn't be severely malnourished.

This wasn't because René was providing more of his paycheck, but it was nonetheless a result of his new job. From his first day working for Mr. B, they told him to bring home food for us. Our children's cheeks had rounded out, and I had more food to eat while I was pregnant because of their generosity.

As my due date was looming, I had to deal with news about the health of Jo-Ann. Since her birth three and a half years earlier, she had dealt with an undiagnosed illness that resulted in pain.

When I had brought up her constant crying at the hospital after she was born, they had told me it was gas. As the months passed and she was still not alright, the doctor said she was just a colicky child. But now, at her last checkup, they had found she had kidney problems and would have to be monitored at the hospital.

The news of having another child with persistent health problems made me wonder what the future would hold if I didn't start making changes. I had always prided myself on being able to manage against all odds, but was it right to keep going against such high stakes?

I was healthy, but I was spent trying to divide attention, time, food and money between my children. It wasn't fair to them, and I decided that this would be my last pregnancy. I asked the doctor if he could perform a hysterectomy after the birth.

Lorraine Patricia Lessard was born on July 18, 1962. My sixth beautiful child. She was a healthy big baby at over 10 pounds. Knowing she was the last of all my babies, I spoiled Lorraine compared to all the others. Susan, my mini-boss watching my lead, also spoiled her baby sister. Everyone knew if you wanted to get in good with me, you had to love Lorraine. She was nicknamed Baby Lorraine by me, a few others called her the spoiled brat. But they were careful to watch how they acted around her when I was there.

Eight months after Baby Lorraine's birth, we moved into the basement of a brownstone on Overdale Street in an inner-city neighbourhood called Little Burgundy, slightly southwest of downtown Montreal. My sister Loy and her family lived upstairs. I struck a deal with the landlord, Mr. Fleming, that would finally allow me to give my children some stability. The landlord's deal was that we'd watch his Great Dane, and he would only charge me $80 a month rent.

Jo-Ann was terrified of the dog. The Great Dane slept in the spare room on a mattress, and the older kids slept in the main room on another mattress. The smaller ones, René Baby-La-La and Baby Lorraine, slept in dresser drawers.

The basement was badly insulated, and ice would form on the walls at night. The basement used to be a bakery, and all the little ovens were still there, along with hundreds of rats. Once again, I would stuff the holes in the walls with broken glass and steel wool; the older kids already knew my methods. They would help me protect us from rats. It was like a tag-team at night. One by one, we would take turns watching the rats as they ate through the steel wool. We'd keep an eye out to spot the one rat who'd be the first to make it through the wool and try to climb up on the blankets. Then it would become a game of whack-a-rat. A stick would usually do the job. Whoever was watching the rats at the time would whack it till it died.

The kids had become my partners, trying to secure our home. They were good kids but being put into that situation created behavioural issues in some of them. Daniel, who was eight years old, became harder to handle. He knew I was stretched out between all of the kids and used it to his advantage to act out. When René would come home, he would have to discipline him often. The other kids would want to watch, but René would say, "Whoever wants to watch gets a spanking too," and they would all scatter. René didn't enjoy having to spank the children. He liked being the fun parent, the one who took you out.

René would often bring Daniel to his brother Dollard's house. It became such a habit that Susan and I would protest. We are a family of six kids. Take all except Baby Lorraine or none. They all deserve a break from the cold and the rats. A few times, he would invite all of us to his mother's for supper. At Mrs. Lessard's house, the children were to sit in another room and were told not to make a sound. It disgusted me to no end, and even though they were getting a good meal, I would rather have them eating with me at home. René's mother treated us like beggars. Keep your food. My children deserved to be treated with respect. Although their clothes were tattered, and their shoes never fit, they were always clean and well-behaved.

"René," I would yell at him, "I will not accept this behaviour from your mother. You can go, but my children are better off with me. How many times was I left in the street with my babies? Nowhere to go, while you were given a warm bed at your mother's and food in your tummy! How selfish you are."

He would leave and not come back for a few days. When he would come back to the house to see the children, he would restart to say that Baby Lorraine was not his. I couldn't take his accusations seriously. This dark-eyed big girl could only be his, dark like Jo-Ann. This was the beginning of what would eventually be the end.

Chapter 14
Stomp

"I'm convinced my cockroaches have military
Training I set off a roach bomb, they diffused it."
- Jay London.

THE BROWNSTONE ON OVERDALE was the first place we had stayed put for longer than a year. I was so proud of having made that deal with Mr. Fleming. Yes, it was badly insulated, had rats and other living beasties, but for once I felt my trunk could be put away in the closet.

Overdale was part of a tough neighbourhood, but that didn't mean that there weren't nice people who lived and worked on the street. Right beside the brownstone, there was a small diner; Jimmy, the owner, was friendly and would allow me to make a few extra dollars clearing out the lunch rush. While clearing the dishes, I would ask the businessmen who ate there if they wanted their laundry washed. "If you want, I'll get that collar really clean and fresh-pressed."

Most of them said yes. I would use my trusty washboard and iron that I hated with a passion, but that came in quite handy to do the job. The laundry combined with babysitting kids would make enough to cover our rent money. I was willing to find as many odd jobs as possible to keep my family together. René was hardly home. He would say he had to be on call at work or needed to visit his mother. Since he wouldn't come home, he wouldn't bring the food from Mrs. B. The food would end up going to his mother's house in those days. Hunger was back in our lives. I didn't let that daunt me. I knew the places that threw out good lettuce and vegetables and would pick through the dumpsters. My pride was gone; I was concerned only with feeding my family. Susan would watch the younger kids so I could work at the diner during the morning before they left for school. Jo-Ann was a picky eater. Susan had little patience, and sometimes she would be mean to get Jo-Ann to eat. Every time I'd step back into the apartment, the kids would be waiting to tell me the stories of how Susan had mistreated them. It was quite loud in the mornings. Susan and I had an understanding. She forced her rules when I was not there.

The younger ones didn't like her rules and made sure to let me know.

For breakfast, when I was there, and we had the ingredients, I'd prepare my specialty, porridge with powdered milk and lots of sugar. The kids loved it, even if the lumps were the size of small meatballs. It has been said I am not the greatest of cooks; actually, one of my children said, "Mommy could burn water." I tried my best, but it wasn't a skill I mastered. My goal with cooking was to make enough for six kids, even if the meal wasn't the most appetizing. For lunch and supper, bread was almost always present. They would share a sardine can with bread between them or bread with sugar and powdered milk or beans on toast. On bad days, the kids had to have mustard and relish sandwiches for lunch. The kids were made fun of at school because of their poor meals. Four out of the six kids were in school. It wasn't easy to ensure they had individual healthy lunches, clean clothes, and their homework done. I felt like I was a candle burning on both ends. I couldn't count on René, and relying on my family wasn't an option. Although my dad seemed concerned about us living in poverty, he never offered any assistance. When he asked me if I was sure if I wanted to marry René and I had said yes, he had told me, "Belle, you made your bed. Now you have to lie in it."

I thought I had glimpsed a softer side to my dad with Susan and Daniel's births, but as we had more babies, the celebrations of the children stopped, and his visits became infrequent. My brother wasn't in a position to help me. He was busy trying to make ends meet for his family. He had five kids and was doing his best to be the father he hadn't had.

At the start of 1965, my loneliness deepened. My sister moved out of the brownstone. She and her husband had decided to settle a little further west, in NDG. Pragmatically, although I had just lost my sister's companionship, my next thought was to talk to Mr. Fleming. I asked if we could move upstairs. He said yes and included the electricity and heating for the same price as we were paying downstairs.

Upstairs, there were fewer rats than in the basement but oddly more cockroaches. Our tag-team whack-a-rat was put to the side for a new activity. Every two months, Jo-Ann, René Baby-La-La, Carol and sometimes Susan, would team up to help me get rid of the roaches. I had a pump spray can. You add water and bleach to the mix, shake it and then when you pumped it, a mist would come out to kill the beasties. "Ok, everyone here? Shoes on? Ready?" They would smile up at me and say, "go, Mommy, go! "I would push the fridge away, and it was like a magic moving floor. Roaches by the thousands, I would pump the spray, and the kids would jump on them as they ran. The kids got a kick out of it thinking they were helping mommy. It made me sad.

I was trying my hardest to bring us up to a level that everyone else takes for granted. The bugs, rodents and the lack of food were only a few of the challenges. The kids were always in ill-fitting clothes and shoes. It's hard to find proper fitting footwear at the Salvation Army. Their teeth were also in bad shape and needed care. I felt that in every way possible, I was not providing enough. It's awful to see your kids not receiving what you feel they deserve.

I didn't know it at the time, but someone was watching and judging my parenting and our poverty.

An unidentified person called social services on us many times. I suspected that it was Mrs. Craig, the supposed friend René had brought into our lives. One afternoon, a woman from the government knocked on my door.

"Mrs. Lessard, we have reason to believe you and your children are not being properly cared for, and the kids are unkempt."

Well, my first instinct was to slap her in the face; I held it in. "Do you have any idea for how many years I have asked for help from government agencies? Your answer was always to get a divorce or separate the children, and we will help." This very stern, tall woman looked at me and said, "Mrs. Lessard, if I decide it, I will take your children from you. If I feel they are in any way, not safe or neglected."

I am not sure what exactly happened after that. I blacked out the rest from my memory. I do know the woman from social services practically ran down the stairs mumbling something about coming back with her superiors.

She returned many times, but the apartment was always clean, and I'd be there to tell her that I did everything for my kids. Eventually, she stopped coming. That's when Mrs. Craig started doing pop-up visits. I think she was trying to catch me doing something elicit, maybe to report to René or the government. Mrs. Craig never realized that I had figured out she was spying on me. If she showed up unexpectedly, I would have so many jobs to do.

"Would you mind watching the children while I do the clients' washing?" Caught off guard, she would be too busy helping me that she couldn't inspect my every move. It gave me a much-needed break.

Mrs. Craig and the social services' surprise visits began to take a toll on me. It's scary to think that someone is spying or checking on you so they can remove your kids.

I felt wound up, and at times my temper was too short, and I took it out on the kids. When I would swat them a little too hard or yell, I would cry in my room afterwards. I would ask God to keep them safe from my misgivings.

I vowed, "I would never separate my children, no matter how bad it gets." As the years would pass, I would realize that saying "no matter how bad it gets" would get pretty bad.

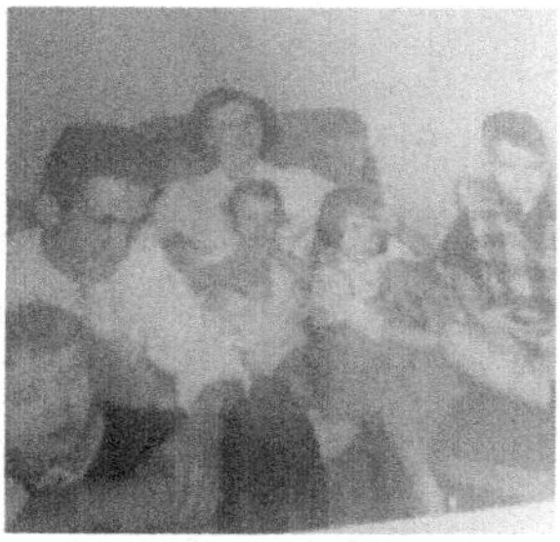

Chapter 15
Nitrous Oxide

"There is no shame worse than poor teeth
in a rich world." - Sarah Smarsh.

OUR DIET, HEAVY ON bread and not much else, played havoc with our teeth. My mouth was in constant pain, and my breath, although I brushed my teeth daily, was pungent. The children's mouths didn't fare much better.

The school noticed, and I was worried that social services would hear of it next and see their bad teeth as neglect on my part.

The idea of having my children removed from my care weighed heavily on my mind. I knew I had to find a way to get them to the dentist.

I made the rounds to the government agencies inquiring about the possibility of getting some help to get their teeth checked and fixed.

I asked if they knew of a dentist who would offer his services as a charity. I was told to go and contact the dentistry departments of hospitals. I picked up my nerve and headed off to the Montreal Children's hospital. Once there, I asked at the reception if I could speak to someone from the dentistry department. A nurse walking by recognized me, "Mrs. Lessard, is that you?"

"Oh, hello, do I know you?" I asked.

"Yes, Mrs. Lessard, I have seen you here many times with your children. I hope they are healthy and doing well." This, I must say, was a little embarrassing. Was I that bad a mother, that a nurse would remember me for spending so much time up at the hospital with my children? "Oh yes, I do recognize your face. Sorry I was just so confused trying to find someone to help me. You've caught me off guard."

"My name is nurse White. Can I help you?"

I thought to myself, go for it, instead of spinning in circles. "Yes, maybe you can. I am looking for some dentist work for my children, I cannot pay, and I wondered if maybe the hospital offers some help?"

"I am sure we do. Let me take you to the dentistry department and see if we can make an appointment."

All medical charges were billed in those days. The truth was I had collected many bills over the years for my children's medical care ranging from my pregnancies, their births and a multitude of illnesses and injuries but had never paid the bills.

I knew I wasn't alone in this; there were many poor people in the same boat as I who couldn't afford care. The doctors had always been understanding of our plight and had never turned us away. If the kids required medication, the doctors would pass me a slip to take downstairs to the hospital's pharmacy. The paper slip would permit me to be given medicine or supplies for free. Doctors took their oath to help seriously, even at the detriment of their pocketbook, but I didn't know if dentists had taken that same oath and would be as forgiving of unpaid bills.

Within an hour, she had set up appointments for the day after for all five children. Baby Lorraine was too young, and I was told they would see her a few years later when she would have her permanent teeth. Early the next morning, my five oldest waited in the hall for their appointments. One at a time, they went in, each for about half an hour to 45 minutes. You get what you pay for, and this was free. The results were dismal. The dentist pulled any teeth that had too much decay and filled the other cavity empty spaces with lead-filled fillings. The procedure was like a factory line, one in, one out. As each child laid down on the chair in the dentist's office, a rubber gas mask was placed over their mouths. One, two, three, and they were out like a light. Pull, fill and get the next child onto the seat until all five are done. I spent the next two days cleaning up vomit and listening to them cry, they were in pain, but I think the vomit was their reaction to the gas. It was awful, but at the same time, I felt good for having been able to get them the help their mouths required.

It gave me the courage to go and find out about my teeth. Many of them were loose because of tooth decay from all the years of poverty, pregnancies and malnourishment. I went to the Montreal General Hospital to find out if I could also get assistance. They gave me an appointment quite quickly.

When the dentist examined my mouth, he told me the best thing he could do would be to remove all my teeth and give me dentures. I was 34 years old and was about to be toothless. The idea made me want to jump out of the seat and run away, but I was still Tuffy Belle; I nodded my head yes. He slid the gas mask over my head, and Tuffy Belle was knocked out cold. There's a taste to the gas that lingers in your mouth once you wake up, and that was about all I had when I woke up. Gums and the acridly sweet taste of knockout gas. I was fitted for my first pair of false teeth. They were to be government-issued dentures, another word for ill-fitting, cheaply made dentures.

I waited impatiently for the dentures to arrive. My gums ached; I would put a cold washcloth on them to try and ease the pain. For once, I was happy that René spent so much time away. I didn't want him to see me like this. I could not bear to look at myself in the mirror with no teeth; I couldn't imagine my husband looking at me and finding me 'Belle' with only gums.

When I went to pick up my dentures, I was incredibly happy. That happiness quickly turned to sorrow when I realized how uncomfortable they were. I felt like crying. Outside of the discomfort, it was a blow to my self-esteem and dignity. One of the things I had always prided myself on was keeping what we had clean and in good shape. Clothes might be used, but they were always washed.

Our furniture right down to our trunk was cared for and dusted. Likewise, when it had come to our hygiene, I made sure my children were washed and that I was always groomed, my hair curled, my nails clipped short, and my teeth brushed. Yet, I had failed to keep our teeth healthy. The loss of my teeth was almost unacceptable, and a source of shame for me.

While growing up, I had regular checkups and dentist visits. My teeth have been straight and healthy. How had I fallen so off? How had I let all my teeth and so many of my kids' teeth be pulled? Would my children have to get dentures as they get older because of the bad choices I made for them so early on?

Poverty had impacted every aspect of my children's lives; no matter how I thought I was protecting them, there was always something that slipped by me to show me I had failed.

Chapter 16

Call Me A Cab

"Oh what a tangled web we weave when we practice to deceive." - Sir Walter Scott. Marmion

ONE MORNING DURING THE summer of 1965, as I was getting Baby Lorraine dressed, I received a phone call at the diner next door. Jimmy sent Jo-Ann and René Baby-La-La, who were playing outside to, "Run upstairs and tell your mom there is a call, quick." I quickly ran down to answer it. We didn't have enough money to have a phone at the apartment, and when people wanted to get a hold of us, Jimmy's diner was the number they called.

"Hello...Hello," I said. "Jimmy, there is no one there?"

Then I heard a cough on the phone, and a female voice answered, "Hello Isabella, you don't know me, but you need to know something."

"Who is this?" I demanded, and the voice said, "Someone who cares. You need to go to the mansion that René works at right now. I know you have struggled with six children, and my heart goes out to you," and she hung up.

Jimmy was staring at me as if I had seen a ghost. The call had sent a bolt through me; I knew whatever I would see at the mansion, it wasn't good.

"Mommy, who was that?" Jo-Ann and René Baby-La-La were both pulling at my dress.

"Jo-Ann, René Baby-La-La, go upstairs and wait for me. Go see Carol." I told them. I was confused. I didn't know what to expect or prepare for, but I knew I had to go there right away.

"Jimmy, I need to borrow ten dollars. Please, I will give it back from my work at the diner."

"No problems, Belle, give it back whenever you can."

"And please, Jimmy, check on my kids and call me a cab."

Fifteen minutes later, I arrived at the mansion. I told the cab to wait. I walked up to the limo parked in the front. René was not there. I didn't want to ring the doorbell, so I went by the yard's side, around to the gardens. I heard whispering and giggles. And then I saw them, standing against the mansion wall. Oh, he was a handsome man in his freshly pressed white shirt and suit. I had spent many hours making sure it was just right for him, scrubbing it on my board until my knuckles were raw and starching it just right. She was not tall, average looking, and she wore a nursing outfit with a nurse bonnet.

René had his hands all over her, fondling her through her uniform as they kissed.

I made a sound, and they both looked, startled, "Belle, Qu'est-ce que tu fais ici?" René asked. She looked at me, mouth gaping. I didn't see her; I saw all the struggles we have been through, the begging on my knees, the rats, the derelicts, the pity strangers gave me, and I saw all my babies' faces hungry, and that fucking trunk. I didn't want to see any more. I turned, and I walked away. René did not bother to follow me, I went back into the cab, and I said, "Please bring me back to Overdale Street."

Jimmy was sitting on the porch, eating Popsicles with the kids. When I got out of the cab, he told them to head upstairs. They fussed, curious to know where Mommy had gone to; I guess a rushed cab ride seemed like quite an adventure for them. "We wanted to see Mommy." Susan saw my face. She knew something had happened and, in her best mini-boss voice, shooed all the kids upstairs as she carried Baby Lorraine up.

"Jimmy, I would like to thank you for all your kindness. Maybe one day I can repay you. But not today."

I started to cry, and the tears were of losing my battle with my marriage. I had made so many sacrifices to stand by this man's side, this adulterer. And I had subjected my children to disappointment after disappointment as I put my marriage before their well-being. I cried for all our empty bellies as we laid cold and hungry at night, while their father was warm and fed at his mother's house. I cried for standing on street corners with six kids with nowhere to go. I cried for begging in churches, at the Salvation Army for a handout, a loaf of bread for my kids. I cried for my kids, I cried for myself, and I cried on my knees for my mother. I need you now, Mom!

Jimmy held me until I was finished. I slowly stood up, trying to compose myself, and I told him in the steadiest voice I could muster, "Thank you."

I went up to the apartment. I picked up Baby Lorraine and kissed each of my children, and I said,

"Daddy won't be coming home. It's our home now, not his."

René Baby-La-la and Jo-Ann started to cry. Susan did not say a word, nor did Carol. Daniel screamed at me, "You are lying!" and ran to his room.

That night when all the kids except Susan were sleeping, I called her into my room, and I told her what I saw today. I cried, and she held me. My Susan, my first-born. My big girl at the age of 11. Since the age of five, I had relied on her more than I had relied on my husband. Susan would watch the kids, help me prepare supper and complete chores. Was it right or fair? I knew the answer in my heart, but I couldn't admit it right now. I needed her support again, telling her things no child should ever hear about their parents' relationship.

"Lord, what have I done to these children?"

I fell asleep holding Susan in my arms, dreaming I was dancing and singing a sweet summer song with Mom. I had not heard her voice in a long time. René didn't come home that night, or the one after that.

It took a few weeks before he showed up at the apartment. Daniel, Susan and Carol were at school. Jo-Ann was sick and had stayed home, and René Baby-La-la was in his room playing.

I was in the middle of changing Baby Lorraine in the bedroom. He entered as my back was turned from the door. I had just lifted Baby Lorraine up onto her feet on the mattress.

"René, you startled me. What are you doing here?"

At that moment, he reached out his arms to Baby Lorraine, and she recoiled backwards on the bed and started to cry. I snatched her up into my arms and told her," It's ok; he won't hurt you."

I guess the natural reaction would be saying, "It's ok, Baby Lorraine, it's Daddy," But in my head, this man had chosen to leave her and our other children fatherless. He had decided to step out of our marriage and family.

"I don't want you to come here to our home and confuse the children."

"Belle, I am sorry you had to find out that way."

"René, please leave. I have loved you from the first moment. I have done everything for you. I have turned away from my family to make this life work and hid from them in shame. I only ask that you leave. I don't want to know what happened. I don't care when or why it happened. Leave our home."

One week later, he appeared with separation papers in hand.

I signed them and told him, " Don't come back here. I will make it on my own, these are my children, and no one will take them from me."

When Daniel arrived from school and found out from Baby-La-la that his father had been here, he asked me, "Why did you make him leave? Why?" I walked away with no way to tell him. Daniel would blame me for his father leaving, and everyone around would feel his anger for years to come.

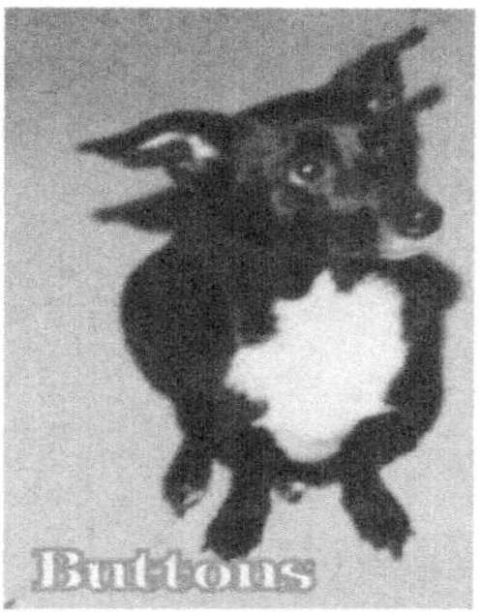

Chapter 17
Puppy Love

"Isn't that the greatest tragedy? When someone rejects us, no matter how they abuse our love we hope against reason that somehow they will come back to us."
- Suzanne E. Anderson.

THE WINTER AFTER I had caught René with his mistress and told him that we were done was a frigid, harsh winter. It was almost like mother nature felt the coldness of my broken heart and decided to represent it in the weather.

The dry cold was tough on Carol; she suffered during the season with a constant croup cough. I kept soup cans filled with water on the radiators to try and keep the air moist. It wasn't enough.

Carol, with her cough, and Jo-Ann with her kidney issues, had to spend endless hours up at the Children's Hospital. Often, I couldn't stay with them. I was pulled in a hundred directions simultaneously; I needed to work at whatever odd jobs were available and still be home for all the kids and yet give individual care to the ones who needed it. I didn't want to give the child protection agency any reason to separate us.

I felt like I was always on the move or watching my shadow.

It was frustrating and affected my calmness. I could see it and felt the switch in my temperament. Before our separation, if the kids acted up, I would have a stern word with them, but their father would do the heavy disciplining even if he did it begrudgingly. Now that was on me. There were instances when I was a little rough when I smacked their bums and regretted those moments. I didn't want to repeat my father's mistakes; my children deserve kindness and love.

René would stop by infrequently to see the children but the older kids thrived on those visits. He had become what he always wanted; a fun dad with little responsibility or obligations towards anyone. He would take them out and never pester them with actual parenting.

Who wouldn't love a man who got you small gifts, sweet-talked you and brought you fun places?

One day in December, he showed up with a puppy, a small, half-crippled, jet-black with a white spot and long like a dachshund puppy.

The kids named her Buttons.

"René, I can't afford a dog. Why would you bring a half-crippled puppy here?"

"Belle, I found her, and I couldn't leave her in the cold. Don't worry. I will fix her leg."

"Bien-sûr René, you will fix it sure," I said, sarcastically.

About a week passed when he returned with Buttons. The kids were so happy. Even Baby Lorraine was excited.

"How did you do it, René?" I asked.

"I threw her into the water, and she swam back and then she seemed better."

"Really René?" I said, incredulously. I was apprehensive about this new responsibility he was about to put on me, yet at the same time, I didn't want to discuss or refute his claim. I just wanted him to leave and go back to his witch.

"The water was freezing; she swam for her life," he said

I couldn't refuse the puppy; she was a survivor like the kids and me. Buttons quickly became Baby Lorraine's little protector. Baby Lorraine would pull her tail, pinch her, sleep on her, and Buttons never left her alone.

The harsh winter wouldn't let up. Soon flu and illnesses flooded Montreal and the hospitals. Baby Lorraine got sick with a fever and a nasty cough. I rubbed her down with camphor oil and made sure the tins on the radiator were full of water. Overnight, her fever started to climb. I bathed her in a cold bath to lower the fever. It didn't. Buttons wouldn't leave her sight. I even stuck Baby Lorraine out in the cold air to clear her lungs, something I had learned to do with Carol. Her fever still wouldn't break and her coughing increased.

I was panicking. I kept calling René but got no answer. Baby Lorraine was getting worse; she couldn't breathe and was at the point of turning blue. By now, the whole house was in a panic.

I frantically called for an ambulance. Thank the Lord for my separation, which had made it that I now qualified for social welfare and that I could afford to get a phone.

The ambulance was my only chance to save my daughter. Susan was pacing up and down the hall. The others were huddled on the couch as I kept praying and rocking Baby Lorraine.

Finally, the ambulance arrived. The paramedic took her from me and told me to come in the ambulance, "she may not make it, and you should be with her." The kids started to cry, and I turned to Susan and said, "You are in charge. I need you to be strong." Susan gathered up her brothers and sisters close to her and huddled back on the couch.

It was like a nightmare. As the ambulance sped down the street, the paramedics worked on my baby, pulling things, inserting oxygen and needles; it was all happening so fast.

"Can I hold her?" and the paramedic said, "She needs you to pray for her, and let us help her."

I started to cry, "Precious Lord, take my hand, Dear Lord, keep her safe."

When we arrived at the hospital, it was a whirlwind; they rushed her into the Emergency room and told me I had to wait outside.

One hour later, the doctor came out and said, "Mrs. Lessard, your baby is resting. A few minutes more and she would not have made it." I almost fainted.

The doctor told a nurse to try and find some orange juice or water for me. He then explained, "your baby had built up too much mucus, and her cough was so great that her esophagus had closed, and she could not get any oxygen to her lungs."

"Is it my fault?" I asked, and he said, "no, these things happen, and I can tell by her size, she is a well taken care of baby.

To help her breathe, we had to open her throat. We then inserted a tube into her lungs to breathe. Once we cleared her throat, we closed the incision and repaired it with a small piece of skin from her ankle. This procedure is done only in the direst circumstances. It's called a tracheostomy. Perhaps you should contact your husband and ask him to come to the hospital," he said.

"Your baby is heavily sedated and will sleep through the night."

I answered that I couldn't reach my husband, we are separated, and I have five kids at home waiting for word on their sister.

With a kind face, he turned to the nurse who had returned with my orange juice and said, "Can you please call a taxi for Mrs. Lessard, give her a few minutes with her child and make sure to give her the money for the taxi, please." When I walked into the ICU room, my eye caught Baby Lorraine's bed right away. She had tubes everywhere and a little blood on her gown. I cried for her and thanked the Lord that she was safe.

As I kissed her forehead, I heard a whimper, and a tear was drying on her face.

The taxi pulled up to our place, and as I got out of the car, Susan whipped open the door, and all the others clamoured out with Buttons in tow.

"Where is Baby Lorraine, Mommy, tell us."

I hugged all of them and said, "She's resting. A doctor saved her life tonight. We will all walk to the hospital tomorrow, so everyone go get some sleep now." When everyone went to sleep, Susan came into my room. "We almost lost her, Susan." Susan and I cried and held each other until we passed out.

A few nights later, my sister-in-law called me up and said, "Isabella j'ai de mauvaises nouvelles." I just rolled my eyes and sat down. "Andrée are you all right?" I asked.

"Of course, bien sûr, mais je suis inquiète pour toi et les enfants."

"Andrée, speak to me in English, so I don't misunderstand what bad news you have."

"Very well, Belle" Andrée never called me Belle. Something must be very wrong.

She continued, "René came over last night to say goodbye to Mother and me."

"Goodbye? Where is he going?" I asked. I still hadn't reached him and hadn't been able to tell him about Baby Lorraine.

"He is moving to Germany."

I was glad I was sitting because this news stunned me; I secretly still loved this man. René never asked for a divorce; it always left me hoping there was a chance that he would apologize and we'd get back together. Wake up, Belle no-no-no. He didn't care about you or the kids he left behind.

"He is going with that German nurse. I also heard some rumours from our brothers that she has a child or two with him... Hello... Hello... Hello... Belle, are you there?" asked Andrée.

"I am Andrée; I am always there." By that, I meant always there in a struggle. "Andrée, I will have to let you go. I have to go to the hospital and pick up Baby Lorraine."

"What happened to Lorraine?" she asked.

"I almost lost her, and if the family reached out more often, you would have known this. I couldn't even reach her father. Now he is gone. So, my sister-in-law, I must go."

Late at night, once again, I cried myself to sleep, one-woman, six kids, no job, alone - I felt so alone.

Susan didn't come to me that night. I wondered why and hoped against hope that the reason wasn't that I had relied on her too heavily and that she too would now leave me.

Chapter 18
Daniel René Lessard

"I'm half good and I'm half bad. My mama is a very good girl and my daddy is a very bad boy. And I guess that leaves me somewhere sort of...here." - C. Joy Bell C.

THE DOWNTOWN NEIGHBOURHOOD of Overdale started to consume my children. The older ones were now going through adolescence. Susan was 13, and Daniel 12. At the cusp of being a teenager, Daniel had many anger issues due to our poverty, his father's absence, and belief that I had pushed his father away.

Not knowing what to do, I would send him to spend weekends with Uncle Bob and Aunt Sonya. They always welcomed him into their home. Uncle Bob tried to steer Daniel on the right path, but Daniel, very much the angry teen, was looking for trouble.

He started to hang out with a boy named Sonny from the top of the street. This boy and his family were bad news.

I had already gotten a taste of the type of people they were because Susan and Carol were friends with Sonny's two sisters. Susan wasn't an angel but could be around bad people without them affecting her, but Sonny's sisters were a mean and destructive influence on Carol. Carol had always enjoyed drama, such as seeing one of her siblings getting in trouble.

However, when she was with Sonny's sisters, she became fascinated with seeing others in pain; they would be the first to arrive at an accident or laugh at someone's mishap.

I was worried when I saw Sonny befriending Daniel.

With six kids and being Tuffy Belle, I kept my children mostly in line; sometimes, all I'd have to resort to was the threat of me shaking my fist at them. It did the trick. I was the boss in the house, and Daniel was a little afraid of me, but once he left the house, I knew I had no control over his actions.

He was skipping school, coming home at all hours, and I had even smelled alcohol on his clothes. I soon started hearing rumours he had experimented with drugs. The more I tried to keep him reined in, the more he acted out. He would tell me how much he resented me for having made his father leave. I was at a loss on how to keep him home and safe.

One day, Daniel was playing on the train tracks with Sonny and some other young hoodlums. Daniel fell as Sonny and the other boys watched and laughed. Daniel came home and went to bed, only to wake me in the middle of the night, in pain and told me what had happened.

I had no money for a taxi to bring him to the hospital. I could only ice his bruises. In the morning, I asked Mr. Craig for a lift to take Daniel to the hospital. He had two broken wrists. This meant he'd have to stay home from school and listen to my rules. Rule one: No Sonny! Three months later, he had healed and was back in the streets with Sonny and the other hoodlums, the Little Burgundy gang. Our neighbourhood was often described as a slum—a description it had earned due to its poverty-stricken residents and its abundance of street gangs. The trouble picked up as if he had never left. He came home, blood pouring from his head and actually tried to hide it! His head had been split open by a rock while they were playing chicken. I found him a lift to the hospital and the money for the 45 stitches.

I tried to discipline him. I ended up breaking so many paddles on Daniel, yet he wouldn't stop. Uncle Bob tried his best to get him to behave, as did Uncle Dollard. Even though René had abandoned us, his brother Dollard never abandoned Daniel. We all refused to quit on him and tried to show him we cared. Unfortunately, my son was hard-headed.

Six months after the rock, he was hit with a frozen beer bottle. Hospital again, and I pleaded with him, "Stop hanging around with Sonny!" It was too late; the damage had already been done.

He moved on to more dangerous gangs from Little Burgundy. Stealing, fighting, and late-night phone calls from the police followed. After one too many of these calls, the police told me to place him in Weredale, a home for delinquent teens. So, I did.

That weekend, I packed up Baby Lorraine and took her to visit Daniel at Weredale. He begged me, "Mom, I'll be good. Please let me come home." I did. I just wanted my Daniel back.

It didn't work. He would end up in the delinquent teens' home again and again. He started running away, the police would find him and bring him back. It broke my heart each time.

Daniel was my child, he had just turned 13, and I was afraid for him and starting to be afraid of him.

The next time he ran away from Weredale, Daniel stole my rent money for drugs and alcohol, and I had no way of getting that kind of money back. I cried again on my knees, and I asked God to help.

I knew I had to make a big decision. I have five other children relying on me.

I called the police. Yes, I called the police on my son. Do you know what that feels like? It felt like fire running in my body; it felt like needles stuck in my eyes; it feels like my heart had no beat. It felt like I failed him. René, you fucker, where are you!

The cops came to my door and asked, "What would you like us to do with him, Mrs. Lessard?" I didn't trust him with the other kids at home; all I could say was, "Take him to Weredale."

I can still see the look of desperation in his eyes. He was pleading for me to let him stay, but this was not my son; this was a sorry version of my Daniel. Drugs and alcohol had taken hold of him.

Every Sunday from that day on, Baby Lorraine and I would go see him. Baby Lorraine would smile at him, and he would look at her, and smile and I would see a glimpse of my Daniel. I would ask how it was here, and he would shrug his shoulders and say, "Alright. Mom, I am truly sorry. I did you all wrong."

A few months later, he was back home. He was seemingly staying out of trouble, which was a godsend because we were about to have our first out-of-town guest.

Loy was up from the States.

She, along with her young family, her hubby Russell and their four kids had moved there for her new job. I hadn't seen my sister since her move. I needed this visit; it felt like a lifeline.

The kids were happy to see her, and she had a surprise gift for them. She had brought them a beautiful puppy. He was a collie mix, just like Lassie. As Loy and I were embracing, the puppy and the kids ran around, squealing along with little Buttons barking at the new puppy.

"Loy, we can't afford another dog."

"Belle, isn't he cute?"

I just stared at her with my mouth gaping open, incredulous that people kept bringing me dogs as if I didn't have enough mouths to feed already.

"Mom, it's Bingo," said Baby Lorraine and I had no choice.

Loy stayed for a few days. We talked and hugged and hugged some more. My baby sister was back in my arms.

Late one night during her stay, Loy and I were having a cup of tea outside on the stoop. The younger kids were all asleep, and Susan had gone to a friend's house. Daniel was out.

A car pulled up and laughing young teenagers were in it, out steps Daniel. Loy and I jumped up and told the teens in the car to get lost, and I could see Sonny was in there.

"Daniel, what the fuck were you doing with them?" I was livid.

I pressed my finger into his chest repeatedly. He just stared at me. Loy said, "Calm down, Belle."

"No, he is going to answer me."

Daniel looked at me but stayed quiet.

"What the fuck were you doing with them?" I was so angry. I was propelling him backwards.

"Belle, keep your voice down now," said Loy.

"Why who cares about my voice, the drug dealers, the pimps, the fucking drug addicts like MY SON!" The fire inside me was burning bright, and I could not control it.

"NO! He is going to answer me! Pull up your pants and smarten up," I was yelling loudly. The last year and a half of having dealt with his misplaced anger, his outburst and constant trouble while I tried to get him the help he required finally made me explode. "YOUR FATHER FUCKED UP! HE LEFT US. HE HAS TWO OTHER CHILDREN! YOUR PRECIOUS FATHER IS IN GERMANY WITH THEM! I gave my best and my life and my dignity to your father! If you can't get over it, too bad for you. I won't quit on you EVER! But I can't keep having you punish yourself and me because of your anger."

I shoved him so hard he fell back. Daniel pushed me to get me off of him, and I stumbled. Loy had seen enough. Daniel would never hurt me, but it scared Loy. Loy opened the door and urged me in. Upstairs she called the police, and Daniel was gone again.

The morning after, Loy was departing back to the States. It was a sombre day. The rain was pouring, and the kids were home from school. Loy spent the early morning apologizing for calling the police. I told her it was destined to happen again, and I just felt like giving up. Loy left, and I was at a loss.

I decided to take a trip up to Weredale. I left Susan with the kids. It was a 45-minute walk and gave me time to think of what to say to Daniel. When he was brought out to the meeting family room, his eyes were red from either no sleep or crying. "Danny." I always called him Danny when I was feeling sorry for him. "I am sorry about last night."

He looked at me, and he didn't say a word. When I got up to go, I said, "maybe I'll come back later in the week, and maybe you will talk to me" as I turned to walk away, I heard him whisper. "I would never hurt you, Mom, not the way he did. I will always protect you and my family. I am your son."

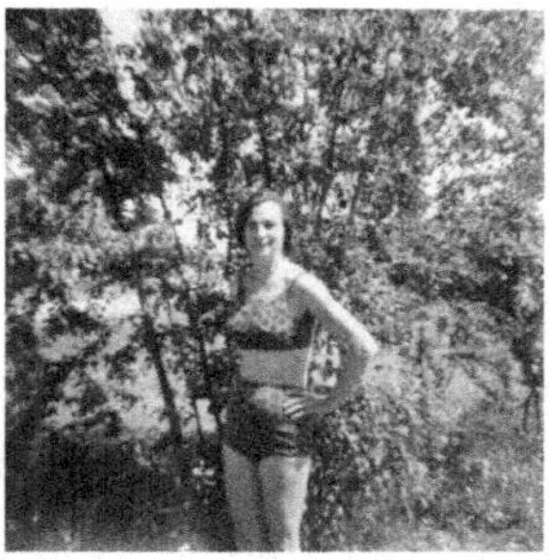

Chapter 19

Lessons Learned

"She is water, powerful enough to drown you. Soft enough to cleanse you. Deep enough to save you." - Adrian Michael.

I WAS A SINGLE MOM on welfare with six kids. Life often felt like it was spiralling out of control. Sometimes all it took was my youngest but my most vocal child to make me lose my cool.

That's what happened on the day that Baby Lorraine wouldn't stop pestering me.

I was on the phone with Rita, a new friend from the neighbourhood.

I was speaking in French so that Baby Lorraine couldn't understand.

"Mommy, speak French to me! Mommy, Mommy!"

"Get lost, Lorraine! Just get lost! Mommy's on the phone." I turned my back to her to try and get some peace.

Baby Lorraine picked up her dog Buttons, put her in the tram carriage, and she left.

She must have been smaller than a pea, but she left. Fifteen minutes later, as I finished my phone call and looked around the living room, I realized it had gotten so quiet because there was no one in the room.

All hell broke loose when I realized Baby Lorraine was nowhere in the apartment. Little Burgundy, with the pimps, prostitutes and street hustlers, she was prey for the sick fuckers. I had to find her quickly. I ran downstairs and into the diner.

"Help, I can't find my baby!" Jimmy called the cops, and I went out into the street, screaming her name hoping she was nearby.

Everyone from the neighbourhood helped me search. I was so worried, I couldn't think straight. I just kept yelling and going down roads hoping to see her.

She was found an hour later, by the police. She was walking with her dog in the carriage a full ten blocks away on Dorchester Street in downtown Montreal at the height of rush-hour. I was incredibly relieved, yet I was dumbfounded. Why did no one ask why is she here? Where are her parents?

When she got home, I told her never to leave without telling me where she was going, and she shrugged her shoulders and said, "Okay, Mommy," and that was the end of that in her head.

But not in mine; I would never forgive myself for putting her in danger because I didn't have a minute for her. This was a lesson on how fast bad things happen but also to always put my children first. There were more lessons to come. We lived in an area that doled them out, quite frequently.

It was only a few days after Baby Lorraine's misadventure that my Jo-Ann and René Baby-La-La were targeted by a deviant. I was upstairs with Baby Lorraine, the older three were out with friends, and Jo-Ann and René Baby-La-La were playing outside in front of the diner. I heard screaming from the window. I ran down the two flights of stairs. A shirtless man with his pants half down was chasing both of them around a parked car. I screamed, "Kids get in the house!" They dashed to the door.

"Hey, do you know whose kids they are, you dirty bastard?"

He was so drunk, I walked up to him, and I punched him so hard in the face, he went down. I went inside, and I called the police. With all the commotion, the whole street, including the diner's patrons and Jimmy, came outside. By the time I got back downstairs, he was gone.

"Where did he go?" and Jimmy said, "don't worry, Belle, he won't bother your kids again."

I trusted Jimmy's word. The two events happening in such a short span made me decide to take all of my kids, including Daniel, away from the city, for a bit.

Daniel was still at Weredale but he was allowed to come home on the weekends. I asked Weredale to give him a special pass so he could join us on vacation.

We were all excited and looked forward to our first family trip. Before going away on the trip, Daniel wanted to relax instead of being under my thumb and roof for the weekend. He went to stay at Mr. and Mrs. Craig's. Mrs. Craig let him go out and do whatever he pleased. Old habits die hard; he went out to meet up with his friends.

They drank and did drugs, and Daniel ended his night being hit by a car. Injured and bleeding, he hobbled away from the accident without getting medical attention; he didn't want to ruin his chances of being let out of Weredale. He tried to enter Mrs. Craig's home. Mrs. Craig told him, "You are bleeding, don't step in my house. You'll stain something!"

Daniel said, "I was hit by a car!"

"If you don't want me to tell your mother, then stay outside until you stop bleeding."

Daniel laid across the steps until the next day.

When he woke up, Mrs. Craig wasn't home, and Mr. Craig let him come in, wash up and clean his cuts.

When I found out, I was shocked by Mrs. Craig's callousness towards a child she had always professed to love. It was another lesson; not all those that come into our lives offering a helping hand should be trusted. Weredale was none the wiser about Daniel's accident and bad choices. He was given his two-week pass to head out on vacation with us.

I was too poor to have planned and paid for a trip away. This vacation had come about because each summer, the welfare office offered low-income moms and kids the chance to go to Macaulay camp, an hour and a half drive west of the city. This would be two weeks of sun, beach and cooked meals, away from Overdale and all of Montreal's problems and dangers.

We gathered at the Church on Atwater street and rode buses to the camp located in Hawkesbury, Ontario. The kids loved every moment; even the bus was an adventure for them.

When we arrived, they gave us our cabin number and our counsellor's name and patch for our group. Each group had a name like the bears, the foxes etc.

The counsellors were there to entertain the kids and give us mothers a reprieve. As the kids played sports, the moms got a chance to do crafts and swim. My friend Rita had also qualified for the trip. She and I would spend most of our days together at the camp, reminiscing about our childhoods and enjoying the pleasures of summer. It felt so good to be able to let our kids experience singing by the bonfire and roasting marshmallows, all the things poor city kids never experienced. On rainy days, kids and moms would congregate in the mess hall, play games, and act out movie scenes.

Rita had four bad kids; I mean, really bad. They were about a year or two older than my Baby Lorraine. One day at the beach, the moms were to supervise the swimming in the St. Lawrence River. Baby Lorraine and Rita's kids were swimming together when I noticed a little head bobbing up and down, but the head wasn't coming out of the water more than to the hairline. I quickly ran in. I can't swim, but I was scared that one of the kids was in danger. It turned out that the head-bopping was my Baby Lorraine's. Rita's youngest son, Timmy, was holding her down by her legs and trying to drown her.

I pulled her out. Baby Lorraine just kept coughing up water. Luckily she appeared to be okay. Rita told me since we shared everything, including the cabin, "Belle, take Timmy up to the cabin, and you punish him as you see fit. "I dragged his little ass up the hill to the cabin, and I beat him on his butt until he'd had enough. I do not regret it. He almost drowned my baby, and he had probably scared her off water for life.

Happily, those bad moments were few and far between. During the two weeks, the kids laughed more than I had seen them laugh in the last year. It was such an amazing feeling to be at ease with my children - a break from the heaviness that had become our lives.

This camp made us all feel free, free of the inner city, of dirty streets and the survival of the tough downtown life. I vowed I would bring them every year.

Chapter 20
New Beginnings

"I salute the light within your eyes where the whole universe dwells, for when you are at that center within you and I am at that place within me, we shall be one."
- Chief Crazy Horse

WHEN WE RETURNED FROM our two-week vacation, I went back to working the lunchtime clean-up at Jimmy's diner. One afternoon, while I was clearing dishes, a tall, dark-haired, tawny-skinned man came in for a bite to eat.

He was handsome. He wore big chunky rings and chains and had a confidence about him. He looked like he may have been a native Indian. He glanced at me and smiled. The diner was frequented by many types of men, from businessmen to blue-collar workers and hustlers. They were all of different races, white, black, and everything in between. Many of them would give me the once-over as I cleared the tables.

These men were mostly married and looking for a casual flirtation. I didn't think much of this dark stranger or how he looked at me; I wasn't looking to boost a man's ego by being his conquest, no matter how good-looking he was. I got on with my cleaning, then went home to the kids.

The next day when I arrived at the diner, Jimmy asked me if I would be interested in going on a date.

I said, "Jimmy, how could you? You are a married man, and I am grateful for your friendship, but I would never!"

He laughed and said, "Not with me, Belle! With him."

I glanced at where he was pointing, and there he was, the mystery man from yesterday. He said the man had asked him who I was. Jimmy had told him not only my name but also about my kids and our struggles. Jimmy said, "And after all that, he still wants to take you on a date. His name is Roger."

When I was growing up as a child, French and English cultures didn't mix, and the races for sure didn't. I had already gone against tradition by marrying a Frenchman. Did I dare go on a date with an Indian man?

Oddly, what made up my mind was an incident that had happened a few years back at Christmas time. Aunt Sonya and Uncle Bob had come over for Christmas Eve supper. The kids were yammering on about Christmas gifts. They asked about nuts using a common North American derogatory slang term for Brazilian nuts.

"Mommy, is Grandpa bringing some n-word toe nuts this Christmas?

"I don't know. I hope he does. Your children just love them."

Aunt Sonya picked up on it. This fun-loving woman got very serious and told me that I should be careful about what I taught my children. My kids were much younger at the time; they didn't know what that n-word meant. And shame on me, I did. I hadn't given a thought to how someone who's not white like Sonya would react to it. She continued, "Racist words grow into racist thoughts, and those thoughts grow into racist minds and actions. Racists have hurt me, and the idea of you being racist distresses me."

She explained, "I was born in Russia, but I was a gypsy. I stood out due to my dark looks and family gypsy traditions. I was degraded and insulted, called half-breed, dirty skin, thief and whore. I moved to Germany for work, yes, but I was also hoping to get away from the daily onslaught of hate. Germany was worse than Russia. This is where those racist words they threw at me became actions. They treated me as if I was a lesser human because of my race. When the war started, they took me captive. The German soldiers passed me around as if I had no value. I love all of you deeply, and it pains me to see the horrible hate that has been passed down to you, Belle. The rest of your family has never accepted me, but you, Belle and your children have always treated me with respect."

I hated having hurt her. Sonya was a shining light whenever she entered a room, and the kids and I adored her. Aunt Sonya was someone I thought of when I contemplated breaking the norm and talking to Roger. By refusing, I could be missing out on a shining light.

I decided to accept my first date since my separation from René.

When Roger picked me up, I had to ask him to wait in the car because Baby Lorraine was attached to me at the hip, not wanting me to go. She was screaming so loud the whole neighbourhood heard her. Susan saved me. She took Baby Lorraine upstairs, where she could still be heard crying. "Mommy, don't leave me! That's my mommy!" It didn't discourage Roger from dating me. He said that my children mattered, as did the bond I had with them, even the one I had with my Baby (brat) Lorraine.

Roger wasn't anything like René.

He seemed reserved on our first date. Instead of sweet-talking me, he asked me questions and reflected before answering the ones I asked; he made me feel heard and safe. I was surprised I hadn't noticed him before; he told me how he worked across the street from the brownstone at Guaranteed Milk and had seen me at the diner a few times. One date led to two, and then more.

As we dated, he opened up to me. Roger was a full blooded Indian. He had been abused by alcoholic parents and had run away at eight years old. He had to fend for himself. Luckily he was resourceful, hunting on the land, finding old abandoned cabins in the woods to sleep in and getting help from whoever would help, be it parents of friends and strangers alike. When he became a teenager, he had found a small job and rented a room. Roger knew what it was like to struggle. We had this in common.

His years of hardships hadn't turned him bitter. He was a kind and generous man. He offered to help me financially, which I refused.

Accepting my refusal but not giving up on helping me, he would bring us lots of fresh milk and milk products. I think it was the first time my kids had fresh milk, not the government powdered stuff, and real butter, not the government margarine, with the colour packet that you had to stir in for it to look like butter.

As our relationship got more serious, I explained that no man would enter my home with my children. I trusted no one with my four girls. He understood that and never tried to talk me out of it. If we were together, it would be at his place, and he would bring me home at the end of the night.

After about a year of dating, the basement of the brownstone became available. I asked Mr. Fleming if Roger could rent it.

Not all places agreed to rent to Indian people in Montreal. Mr. Fleming wasn't like most people. He was happy for me and agreed right away; he said he was concerned about me living alone and was delighted that it wouldn't be the case anymore.

I would go into the basement and stay with him in the evening. Baby Lorraine was okay with me going downstairs as long as I came back before bedtime. Roger loved the kids. He would take us all out for Sunday drives and excursions to beaches, Indian reserves, and car races. During our Sunday drives, when I wasn't looking, the kids would whisper, "go faster, go faster," he would screech the tires and get a kick out of the giggles in the back. They were growing fond of him. Jo-Ann was especially close to him.

He had proven himself to her a few months back; the doctors told me she required surgery due to her kidney condition. During her recovery, he had been there for her and now she was in his corner, loving him.

Baby Lorraine was Baby Lorraine, cautious and slightly bratty towards him. Daniel had a special relationship with Roger. Roger and Daniel shared a love of classic cars, and would spend afternoons talking about them. Carol, Susan, and René Baby-La-La were more reserved, but were beginning to rely on his presence. I was happy, as were my kids, but the house rules didn't change. He was downstairs. We were upstairs.

One night after bedtime, I heard a thump on the floor. I was alone in the apartment with the three younger kids, and they were supposed to be asleep. Daniel was at Weredale. Susan and Carol were spending the night out with friends. I got up and checked all the bedrooms.

I saw a light under the bathroom door; it looked like it was from a flashlight. At first, I thought it was Daniel who had sneaked in from the fire escape; he could get in through the bathroom window that way." Daniel, is that you?"

No answer. I ran into my room and took out my gun. If there was one good thing, René left me; it was the 45 Colt pistol from years ago.

I was nervous, but not scared. The door flung open, and there stood the biggest man I had ever seen. I cocked the gun, and he backed up into the bathroom.

I said, "You better run. I'm going to shoot you!" He ran backwards and jumped out to the fire escape.

I shot him as he was running, right in the leg.

The kids were up now and screaming. Jo-Ann and René Baby-La-La were asking each other, "Is that a real gun?" and, "no, Mommy doesn't know how to fire a gun" and asking me, "Mommy, what is happening, and where did you get the gun?"

"Go back to your rooms! I will tell you tomorrow."

Roger was pounding on the front door. I rushed to open it and flew into his arms. "Belle, what happened?"

"Call the police. I just shot a man who was in my bathroom."

"No, Belle, no police. Where did you get the gun? Is it even registered? If he dies, you will be accused of murder, no police Belle." I calmed down and decided he was right. I'd never asked René where he had gotten the gun. I hoped I hadn't killed the man. At breakfast the next morning, the kids were in awe.

"Wow, Mommy, you really shot him!" They thought I was a hero. I wasn't. I was a single mom who was fearless about protecting her babies. As the weeks passed, and we heard nothing about a man dying from a gunshot wound, life returned to normal.

Roger had been right; no police.

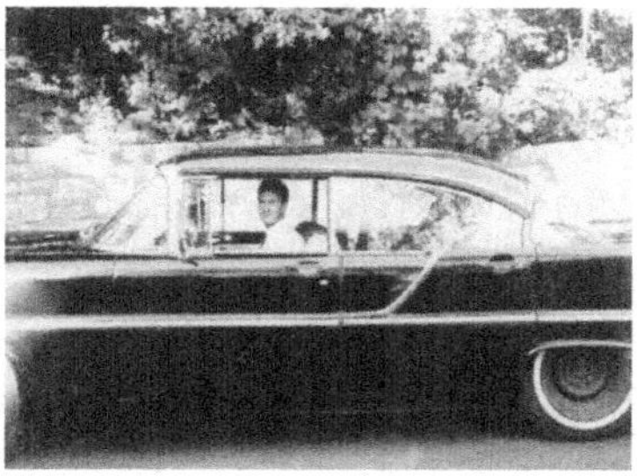

Chapter 21
Decisions

"To forgive is to set a prisoner free and discover that the prisoner was you." - Lewis B. Smedes.

DURING THE SECOND WEEK of June in 1967, a few months after Roger had moved into the brownstone, and I finally felt in charge of my life, the rug was pulled out from under me; by a caller who came to my door. Jo-Ann got to it before me.

"Didn't I tell you to ask first before opening the door?" I yelled out to her. She didn't turn her head towards me. She continued to stare at the caller. I took my eyes off of her and lifted them to the man standing in the doorway.

"Hello, Belle, and you must be my Jo-Ann?"

Jo-Ann, mouth open, rushed off to call everyone, saying, "I think it's Daddy at the door!"

"Can I come in?" he asked.

I was in shock. René was the last person I had pictured ringing my doorbell. I wanted to jump in his arms and, at the same time, close the door on him. I let him in. "Yes, yes, of course."

We went into the living room, and he sat down. In his smooth English, he said, "I've come back. Can I now come home?"

Jo-Ann and René Baby-La-La were standing in the doorway of the living room.

René said, "Is this my big boy, René? Come over here and give me a hug, the two of you." Both kids stood there without moving forward. After a few awkward moments, I told the kids it was okay if they didn't want to hug him. I told them to go to their room and watch over Baby Lorraine.

"René, you have been gone for years, too much time has passed, too many things have happened. Too much, René. I would have appreciated it if you had called before you came."

He looked older, and yet, the same, as if he had never left. He looked like my René.

"Belle, I would like to be forgiven."

"René, I don't know, give me some time." My mind was racing. How dare he show up on my doorstep? I had heard he had two children with this woman; did he desert them also? No, he has to go. We have made it this far; we do not need him anymore. I am the mother, and I am the father. "René, what about your girlfriend? I heard you have a son and a daughter with her."

"Belle, they stayed in Germany," he responded.

I couldn't believe he had done it to someone else. "What are their names?" I don't know why I asked; nothing good could come of knowing.

He hung his head and said," You will never know them."

How sad I felt, not for the woman he had left me for, but I felt an overwhelming sadness for his other children. Didn't René understand how awful it was for kids to lose their father due to his whims?

"I know this is a shock for you, Belle, but I want you to forgive me. If you let me, I want to come home."

As he got up to leave, I said, "René wait, I don't know if I can forgive you or if I want you to come home. I have someone now. His name is Roger, and he has been a support for me in the last few years. Before that, it was your children going at it alone with me. If you would like to see them, you call first, please, and I will make sure they are ready to go with you, but you will bring them home." I couldn't believe I had just said that. Although I felt incredibly shaky, I felt proud for not having given in to him.

He looked at me pensively. He came up to me and kissed my cheek and said, "Belle, I will always love you, and I will wait for your answer, for however long it takes."

He turned and left, and I ran after him to say, "Wait, this is the phone number, be sure to call first." When I got back into the apartment, I crumpled onto myself. What was I going to do? Roger? The children? How could I not accept my husband back, yet how could I take my husband back after all he had done?

By evening all the kids were home and aware that their father had stopped by the apartment. Even Daniel, who half the time couldn't be found because he was out carousing in the streets, was home for supper and to question me.

"Mom, Dad was here?"

"Yes, Daniel, he will call to see if any of you want to see him. He will pick you up and bring you back. Let me know if you want to see him. The only one who I won't allow to go is Baby Lorraine. She stays here."

He looked me deep in the eyes, like his father had earlier that day. As I looked back into his, I saw a glint of happiness for his dad's return. Daniel still blamed me for having pushed his father away. How would he feel if he knew I might refuse his dad's offer to come back home? Would he start to hate me? Would he act out even more? The anguish I felt as I tried to decide on my family's future had me strung out.

René called the next day. Daniel and Susan went to see him, but Jo-Ann and René Baby-La-La would not go; they said they didn't know him. Carol refused to see him. She remembered the birthday when he raised his voice and said, "You wasted money on her, and she isn't even mine." It was a heartbreaking birthday for Carol.

The day passed slowly. I wanted my two oldest at home. I wanted to hear how they felt, how their father was and where they had gone. They came back early in the evening, both of them in good spirits. Daniel told us that René was now working as a warden at the Montreal General Hospital. Had René changed? Maybe he wanted to prove to me that he would be a better father and husband?

I knew I couldn't hide this from Roger. He deserved to know. That night I went down to the basement. I told

Roger about René's return and how confused and conflicted I felt.

Roger listened. He didn't interrupt or say a word until I finished. Reflective, he told me, "Do what your heart says is right, and then you must live with it." He didn't want me to have regrets. I felt secure in his thoughtfulness and love, but I still wasn't sure what my heart was telling me to do. I had spent years hoping for a forever-happy home with René, this could be my one chance, or it could be my downfall.

Roger gave me his hand to hold and told me that he would be there while I took the time I needed to make the right decision. How could I think of leaving Roger, who provided security and love, for a man who hadn't been there consistently for our children and me?

Chapter 22
The Man And His World

"Teach me how to mourn, mother, heal my heart so that I can see the gift of yours that can live through me." - Prayer for healing, Unknown.

THE WEEK AFTER RENÉ'S return passed quickly. Daniel had been sent back to Weredale; he had been caught drunk and causing trouble a day after visiting his father. Susan had been busy bussing tables at a local coffee shop and helping me at home with the kids. She hadn't made another attempt to see her father that week, she said, due to her hectic schedule.

I worried that the real reason was that she hadn't wanted to see him because of what I had told her. I had confided about her father's wishes and my doubts. Susan had become more than my daughter over the years; she was my confidante.

I didn't know if it was fair to her, but I had needed to share the jumble of thoughts going through my mind; unfortunately, sharing it hadn't lessened the turmoil I felt. I tried to keep myself occupied to avoid thinking of it.

No matter how hard I tried, I failed; I couldn't think of much else but René. I was wound up.

Roger gave me space, but he saw how tense I had become with every passing day. He wanted to let some joy shine into our lives; he purchased tickets for us and the younger kids to go to the World fair that Montreal was hosting known as Expo 67, Man and His World.

The kids were so excited. Daniel couldn't come because Weredale wouldn't give him a pass, and Susan said she preferred to work a shift at the coffee shop. I wasn't going to let their absences, René's return, or my mixed emotions deter me from going. I needed a break from real life, and Expo 67 offered just that. Expo 67 was said to be a glimpse of a future utopian city. On Monday, June 26, 1967, I woke the kids early and got them ready, with Susan's help. I had packed lunches the night before. Roger knocked on the door, and we set out. To get to île Sainte-Hélène, where Expo 67 was taking place, we had to take a bus and then the metro (the subway). Taking the metro was a thrilling experience in itself. I hadn't had the chance to go on it many times since it had only been inaugurated the year before.

As we got closer to the grounds, the smell of popcorn, hot dogs and cotton candy was in the air. It made our stomachs growl with hunger even though we had had hearty porridge for breakfast. Only when we reached the entrance, did I realize how big the fair was; Man and His World was huge. There must have been a few thousand people waiting to enter. It was exhilarating to be part of it. The fair had been on for the last couple of months, but this was the first time I could go. The buildings were futuristic and took my breath away. I had heard so much about it but could not picture how amazing it would be; there were glass buildings, triangles ones and one that looked like a giant see-thru dome.

Some minirails went around the fair and dropped you at the different pavilions where the exhibitions were located. To ride would cost us 50 cents per person; Roger said it would be a must, and we got in line. The kids loved it. As we went through the different exhibitions, I allowed myself to fall into the magic of the day. I was looking forward to seeing the kids' reaction to the children's exhibition. Their eyes had been wide with wonder throughout the day, and I knew that one would be the best to end our visit. But first, I wanted to go by the Place des Nations, where the flags represented in the fair were flying, and a show was about to start. Just as we were settling in to hear the anthem, a loud intercom announcement was heard: "Mrs. Isabella Lessard, please come to the reception desk right away; there is an emergency."

My mind jumped to Daniel and Susan. Has something happened?

We pushed through the crowds to make our way, just then the music started, and everyone was clapping. I was worried, and my only thought was, I hope my babies are okay.

We got to the reception desk, and they handed me a phone. As I took the call, I fell to my knees and sobbed. Susan and Daniel were fine, but while I had been enjoying Expo 67, my René had collapsed from a major heart attack at the hospital during his shift and died. René's emergency contact number listed at the hospital was his sister Andrée's. They reached Andrée, who knew of our plans to attend Expo 67. The kids cried because I was crying, and we were taken to a private room and given water. The staff was very kind and took the children to watch the events of Place des Nations on a TV. They wanted to give me time to compose myself. It had been exactly one week since René asked me if he could come back home. I felt numb; I was in shock.

We were driven home by a staff member from the Expo. Once home, I left the kids with Susan, and Roger took me to the hospital to identify René's body. I didn't want Roger there, but he insisted. As we entered the hospital, they brought us into a room where René laid in the bed. He looked peaceful, as if he was sleeping. How could he be gone? It took all of me to keep standing upright. I felt drained of all my blood.

The doctor entered the room and told me they had done everything for him, but his heart valves were blocked, and his heart wasn't strong enough to handle the stress. That's when I learned about René's heart condition, which is why the Air Force years ago had given him the honourable discharge.

I asked for a moment alone, without the doctor or Roger. I needed to be alone with René. As they left, I went nearer to the bed, wanting almost to lay beside him. I needed to touch him, to hold him, to tell him, "René, if you had just stuck around a little longer, I was going to follow my heart and take you back. Why couldn't you wait?" I stroked his beautiful black hair, and I kissed his cheek. I traced the scar on his chest from his terrible fall years ago on the picket fence. I had traced it many times late at night as I watched him sleep. I didn't remember the pain that loving this man had caused me. I only remembered the joy and laughter we had shared. He was my Frenchman. His heart could never have belonged to someone else. How could he desert me again after just coming back?

After leaving the hospital, I asked Roger to drive me to Weredale. "Belle, you need to go home and let all your emotions go," he said. "No, Roger, Daniel needs to hear it from me, and Daniel needs to come home and be the man he should be."

The warden went to get Daniel, and when he saw my face, he said

"Mom?"

"Daniel, Dad is gone," I responded. "Go get your things. You are coming home."

Daniel didn't say a word the whole drive back. When we got home, he went to his room and smashed everything. Susan and Carol stayed in their room, and Jo-Ann and René Baby-La-La went and sat outside until dinner. Baby Lorraine didn't know what was going on, she was only five, and the idea of explaining how her father had just come back and then died was too much for me. I didn't want to tell her, so Susan did and bathed her that night. Daniel didn't come down all evening. Later, when everyone was in bed, I checked on him. He was sleeping.

Alone in my room, I let everything flow out. I cried. I screamed. I kicked, and I punched my pillow.

I was angry at the situation and everyone; myself, Roger, René, even the doctor unable to save him.

I was sad, so very sad. I said out loud, "Alone again, just us."

As usual, Susan came to me, and we both cried until we could cry no more. "Susan, I was going to take him back. Why did he leave? Why?"

In the morning, I managed to call everyone we knew. Andrée and her brothers were very helpful with the funeral arrangements. René's funeral and burial were held in the East End. The day was long. René's aunts, uncles and cousins all came to kiss and hug us, most of them strangers to my children because they chose not to know us when René was alive. One of them scooped up Baby Lorraine to hold her on their knees as they sat. She let out a scream that let them know a show of comfort from a stranger was not okay for her.

Seeing the fuss that she was causing, Mr. and Mrs. Craig took Baby Lorraine, Jo-Ann, and René Baby-La-La to the Woolworths store across the street for hamburgers and milkshakes.

They stayed with them until after the burial and brought them home. That night, I looked at our six beautiful kids that René and I had made. I loved René for many things but blessing me with them was the reason he would always hold my heart no matter the anguish he had caused.

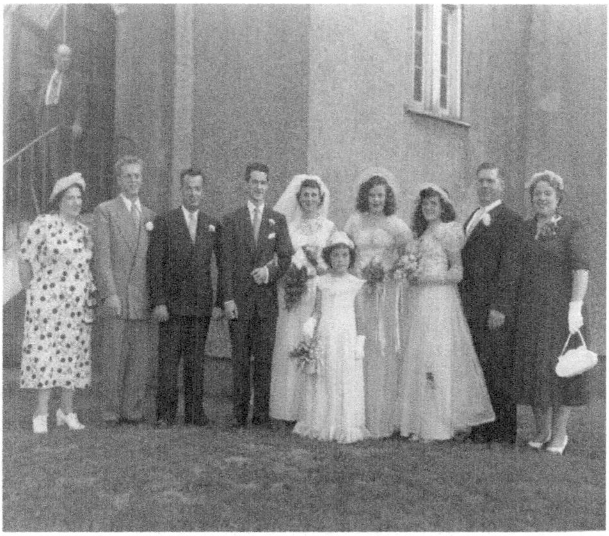

Picture 1: Wedding of Belle Lawrence and René Oliver Lessard, July 5, 1952. Left to right: Mrs. Marie Lessard , Unknown Figure, Dollard Lessard, René Lessard, Mrs. Isabella Lessard, Flower girl cousin Helene, Marion Johnson, Loy Lawrence, Albert Lawrence, Josephine Lawrence.

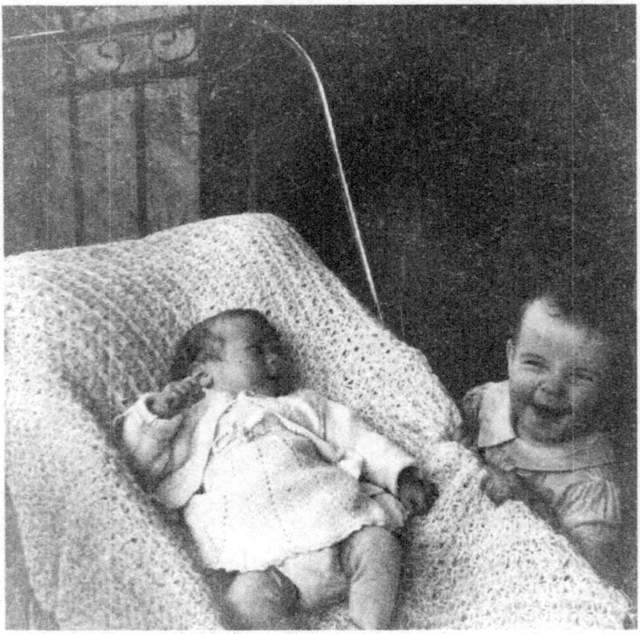

Picture 2: Daniel Lessard, with big sister Susan in 1954.

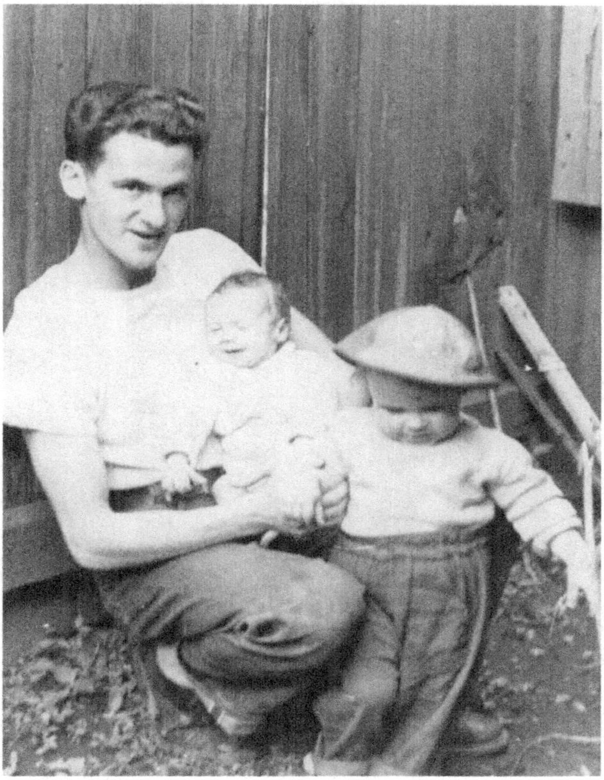

Picture 3: René with Daniel and Susan back of the rooming house in 1954.

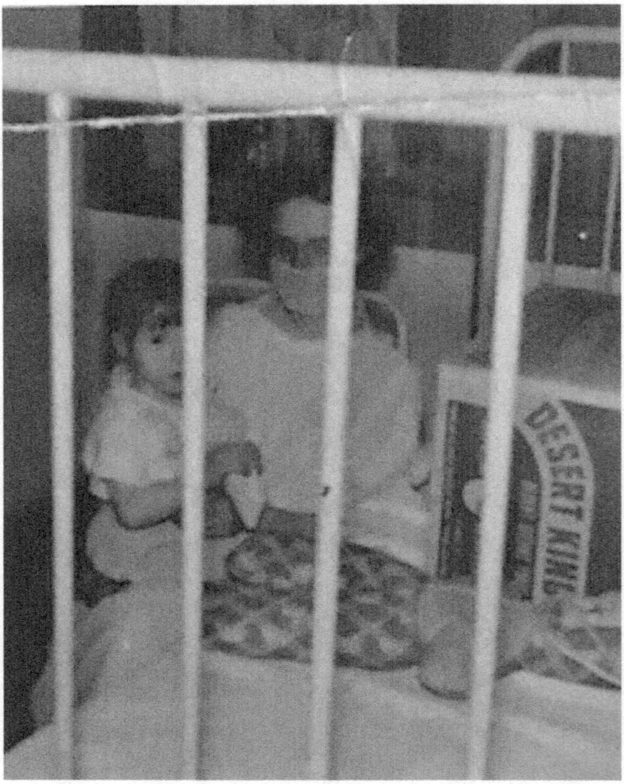

Picture 4: Carol and Belle at the Institute for Diseases in 1957. Carol remained there for two years with Tuberculosis.

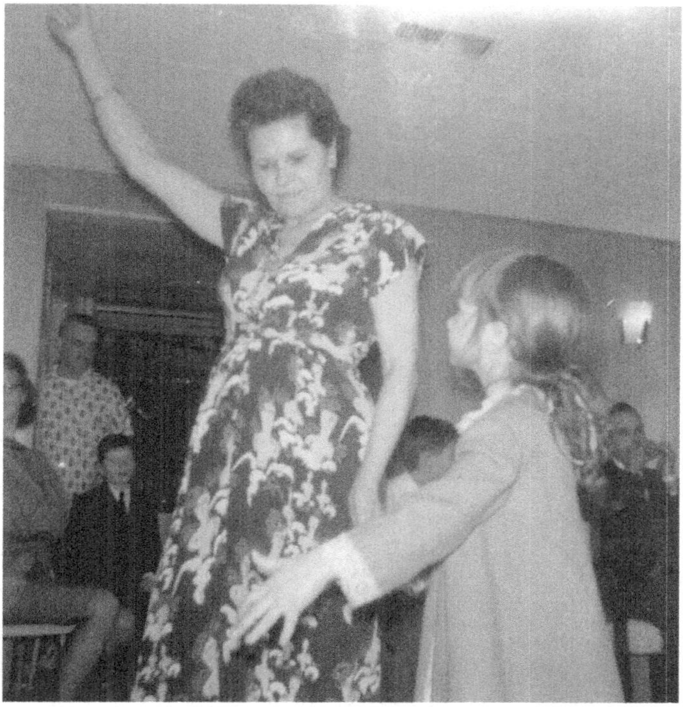

Picture 5: Auntie Sonya always the life of the party dancing with Baby Lorraine in 1965.

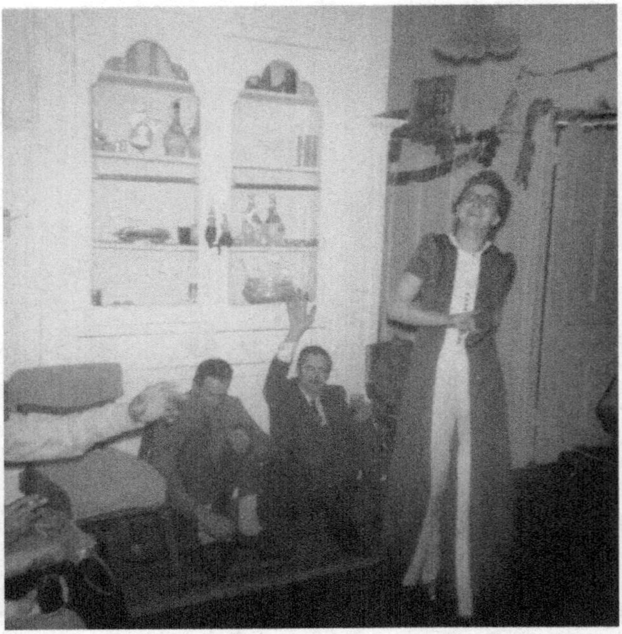

Picture 6: Belle dancing at Christmas with Roger and Bernard in 1974.

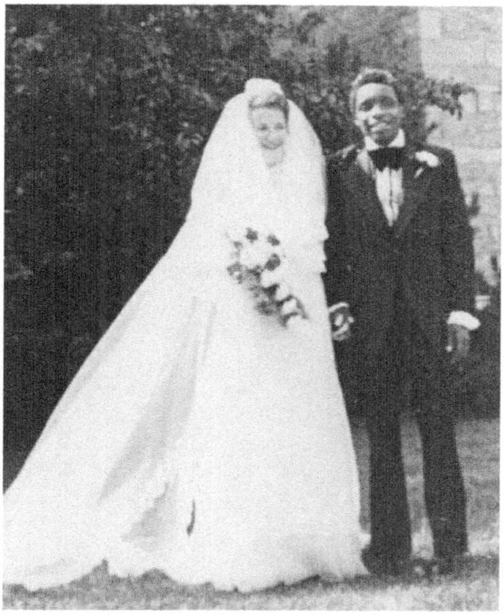

Picture 7: Susan and Peter's Wedding in 1975.

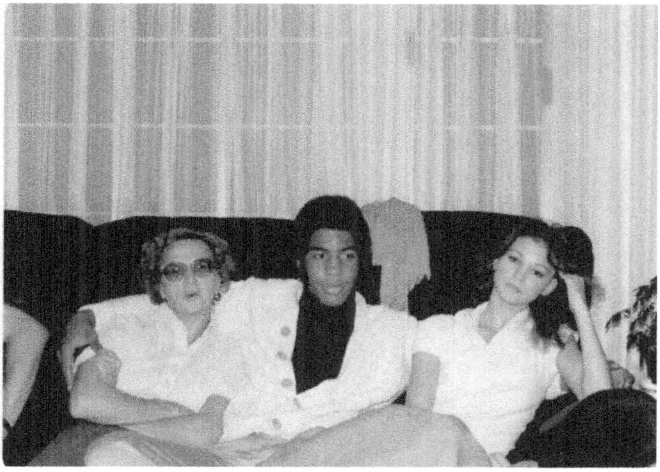

Picture 8: Belle, Darrell, Lorraine at Jo-Ann and Stephen's for Thanksgiving dinner in 1981.

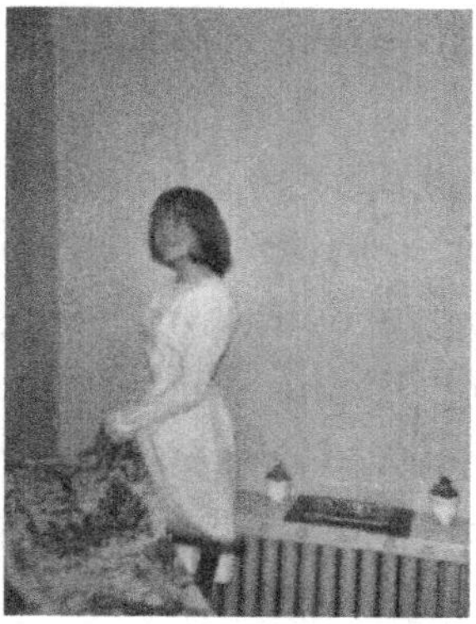

Chapter 23
Always Drama Times Six

"Never regret yesterday. Life is in you today and you make your tomorrow." - L.R. Hubbard.

ROGER KEPT HIS DISTANCE for a long time after the funeral, checking in on us but never imposing or asking me to go downstairs. The first few weeks after René's passing, I was a shell of who I had been. I depended heavily on Susan while I stayed mostly in my room, not knowing how to process René's return and sudden death.

The children following my sombre lead hung around the house. The only ones who weren't morose were our dogs Bingo and Buttons, who provided comfort to the children. As the weeks became months, the pain of loss dulled. I couldn't keep hiding away. My children needed me present, and I needed it too. The kids went back to school in September, and the routines of our lives took over.

Daniel didn't go back to school; he dropped out and started working at a garage. When he was home, he would mostly hang around with Roger and work on cars. At the age of 13, he was the man of our house, although he still required me to swat him at times.

But he wasn't the only one keeping me busy. Carol had just started high school. I don't know if it was because of who she was hanging out with or just because she felt she had to prove herself; she began getting into physical fights with classmates. Most of the time I spent with Carol was because I had gotten word of a brawl, or I had to take her to a doctor's appointment. Jo-Ann, my other beautiful daughter with an illness, would often have to miss school because she was feeling sick. Her surgery a year back had helped but had not stopped her kidney problems. Alone she was very little trouble but combined with her younger brother; they would keep me on my toes. René Baby-La-La was quiet but sneaky. Jo-Ann and René Baby-La-La would team up to play mean spirited pranks on Baby Lorraine. When Baby Lorraine came to me and said they were pulling pranks on her, both of them would get smacked. Baby Lorraine figured that out fast, and sometimes she would make stuff up to get them in trouble. Baby Lorraine, now five, was a spoiled brat. But all of them united didn't come close to the trouble my eldest daughter, my confidante, started to put me through.

Susan had become a master at hiding her real self from me. I had always relied on her to help me, and in that way, she continued to be her old self. But my mini-boss was at an age where she wanted to try out her wiles; at 14 and a half and standing at five foot two, she was all chest and attitude. I had ears and eyes all over the neighbourhood, and that's how I got word that my daughter was pulling a fast one on me. Every morning Susan would leave for school in a proper outfit, and then once she'd get to Montreal High School, she'd change into an outfit that would get her kicked out of class. She must have been hiding a micro miniskirt and a string camisole inside her bag. Miniskirts and shirts with no sleeves were not allowed in school. My mini-boss was never one to let the rules stand in her way. Instead of coming home, she would hang out in her revealing outfit at the place she bussed tables called The Bus Stop.

The one who tipped me off was a prostitute. She had spotted Susan and a couple of her friends at The Bus Stop a few times during school hours and had come by the diner to let me know. It's one of the perks of befriending people no matter their walk of life; you get all the gossip. After getting news of her trickery, I blew up on her. I knew yelling and whooping her wouldn't stop her, but I had to do something.

Susan's two best friends Jocelyn and Marilyn are the ones that would skip school with her. Even though I knew they were getting into trouble, I encouraged her to bring her friend's home so I could see what type of people they were. As I got to know them, I liked them. Jocelyn was a beautiful girl with a lot of character, and Marilyn was sweet and had long hair; she used to come over to iron it on my ironing board.

Both of them were always polite when they stopped by, which was probably more often than when they went to school.

But skimpy outfits and missed school days were to seem like a walk in the park to what was to come early next spring.

One night in March, when the kids were sleeping, I heard noises that sounded like muffled sobbing. I went and checked the kids' rooms and found Susan crying." What is wrong, Susan?"

She turned and looking straight at me said, "I'm pregnant, mom."

I hadn't expected that. I had to remind myself to breathe. After a few minutes, I asked, "How?"

"I have been seeing a guy named Gilles. We made love, Mom. What am I going to do?" she asked through whimpers.

I was shocked. I left the room, and went into mine, and cried, "What the fuck! Am I so bad a mother? What, what, what?" When I got my head together, I called Susan to me, and I told her we would figure this out in the morning.

I pulled Susan out of school after a long conversation with the principal. We both agreed it was the right thing to do. When we got back home, I sat Susan down and started to question her. "Who is this boy ?" I asked.

"His name is Gilles, Mom."

"I already know that. You told me last night. Does he go to Montreal High?"

"No, Mom, he doesn't go to school. He's a biker," she said.

"A biker?" Well, shock number two, I didn't see this coming.

"Yes Satan's Choice Gang."

My mouth dropped open; not just a biker, not just a biker gang, an international biker gang, fuck!

"Susan, he's a criminal. I'm calling the police."

"No, I was willing, Mom. I'm sorry it all happened so fast. I think I love him."

"I can't believe it. He will have to take care of this!" I screamed.

"He can't, Mom. He was sent to jail last week," she whimpered.

I couldn't afford another mouth to feed. We were scraping by; René had left us in debt. But more than that, this isn't what I wanted for Susan.

"Susan, you are too young. You already know how much we struggle because we are poor. But we don't have abortions either. You will carry this baby, and no one will know. Not even your brothers and sisters. When you start to get too big to hide it, you will stay with Aunt Sonya and Uncle Bob. They are the only ones we will tell."

Susan nodded her head, yes. She looked so very young; I wanted to make it all disappear.

When the time came that her belly couldn't be hidden, I made the call to Uncle Bob. The other children missed her but figured she was sent away because she had misbehaved. They didn't ask too many questions. Early that winter, I received a phone call from

Bob. He said it was time. He was taking Susan to the Montreal General Hospital.

I took a taxi. I held Susan's hand all through it. A big beautiful boy was born, and we only had a moment's glance - a nice couple had already arranged to adopt him. Susan and I cried together. When we went home, we never talked about it again.

The father never knew.

Chapter 24
Christine

"There is no denying that there is evil in this world but the light will always conquer the darkness."
- Idowu Koyenikan.

SUSAN DIDN'T RETURN TO high school. She enrolled in a program that would permit her to work in an office or a bank. She had gotten her figure back quickly, which allowed her to dress up in all the cool clothes she desired. Susan had always been a sharp dresser. It made me happy to see her go back to caring about fashion, being young and carefree.

On the outside, she appeared the same as all the other teenagers around her. Inside, though, she seemed more sensitive and alert to things that weren't right. She also knew I was in her corner, and would protect all her secrets, and would help out whenever I could.

She came to me and asked if I could help one of her friends who was stuck in a bad situation. She confided in me about what her friend had had to endure. Her friend's name was Christine. Christine had a mother who was a prostitute with a drug and alcohol problem.

When her mother was high, she would pimp her daughter out to her Johns to get more money for drugs. There was more. Her mother would physically abuse her; she would burn Christine's hands with a hot iron. Susan wanted to know if she could bring Christine here. I nodded, yes.

The following night Susan came home with her. Christine was filthy from the top of her head to her feet. Her clothes stank. The first thing I told her was that she could stay with us until things die down at her mother's. The second was that she needed a bath.

I ran the water and told her to get undressed and get in the tub. Christine looked at me, suspiciously. I said, "If you don't get in, I will throw you in. The rule is you have to get clean to stay here." As she undressed, I flinched. It took everything I had not to gasp. She was covered in razor cuts, whip and burn marks. I saw the iron imprint on her hands. I felt so bad; I had to leave the bathroom.

I told Susan to help her, change the water often, get her some clean clothes and put the other clothes in the garbage immediately after. I cautioned her. "Susan, don't say a word when you see her body. Just clean her and be gentle."

I went into my bedroom, and I punched my pillow over and over again. I swore up and down that if I ever saw Christine's mother, I would put her in the hospital and then call the police.

I believe monsters live among us; I believe sometimes they are in the form of a man, a woman, or sometimes even a child. I know the mother of Christine was no mother at all. She was a monster that lived down the street.

I have seen some horrible things but never have seen a beautiful young girl so marked by the abuse over her young life. I prayed, and I prayed this monster would die.

Christine often stayed with us, and each time she knew to head to the bathroom to bathe before she came to our table and slept in our beds. After the first night, I called the police on her mother. I did it every time Christine would stop by with new signs of neglect and abuse on her body. Christine finally told me her mother knew it was me. She said it made it worse when she went home. So I stopped calling the police, but I didn't stop praying to God for that monster's death.

As time passed, she came by less and less. She would pop in every six months or so. She was evasive of where she lived now and what she did for work. I didn't ask too many questions; my home, the brownstone, was a safe place for whoever needed it in the neighbourhood. I lived by the motto, a poor person doesn't call another poor person poor, they give to the other person. The kids ended up bringing other friends who needed help or animals they rescued; all of them were welcomed into our home, be it for an afternoon, a night or longer.

That was the way it stayed for many years.

Until 1970, the year Mr. Fleming passed away, and the building was sold. The new owners were going to renovate the upstairs, and we would have to move as soon as our lease was up. Roger would get to stay in the basement since they were only renovating the higher floors. I was going to miss our home. It was the longest I had lived anywhere with the kids, and the first place we never got kicked out of. My trunk had remained in the closet for ten years. I told myself that it would stay there when we left. A constant reminder of a life that is no longer welcome. I went to Mr. Fleming's funeral with

Susan. I wanted to pay my respects for the security he had allowed me to give to my young family. He had kept his word over the years and never raised our rent. He had also allowed Roger to rent when some owners would have turned him away. Those simple acts have made such a difference in my life.

When we entered the funeral home, all eyes were on us. I felt awkward. I was out of place. An older, well-dressed woman approached us and introduced herself. She was Mr. Fleming's widow. She told me that her husband had been happy to have us in the brownstone at Overdale. At first, because I took good care of his Great Dane, but after because he thought I was a good mother and appreciated the life I was trying to provide for my family.

Susan stifled a cry, and I hung my head and said, "I have been blessed along my way with good people. Your husband was one of those people. God bless you all." It was a beautiful service for a man who had a kind heart. Once the service had ended, Susan and I went home to pack.

I was unsure where to move. My family was a downtown Little Burgundy bunch, but I felt it was time to live in a safer area.

Susan was 17 and working at the Bank of Montreal (BMO). She would help pay the rent, as would Daniel. He was working as a mechanic. There was also another small push to leave Little Burgundy; Jimmy was retiring. I couldn't imagine the diner without him there. He had given me the chance to make extra income and had even over the years convinced his patrons to provide me with a washer. He was more than a boss.

Before all the boxes were packed, I stood in my bedroom alone and wrapped my arms around myself. I looked out the window and remembered all the nights I stood here waiting for René to return, waiting for Daniel to get home safe, the years of Susan and I crying ourselves to sleep and the sweet breeze carrying my mom's voice to ease my fears and pain. I said a quiet prayer to myself, "Belle is my name, not Isabella, not Isa and not Bella. I have survived this far, and I, Belle, will always be in the mix. I'm my mother's daughter, and she wouldn't want me to be any less than who I am." I closed the door to my bedroom, where I had spent many nights alone.

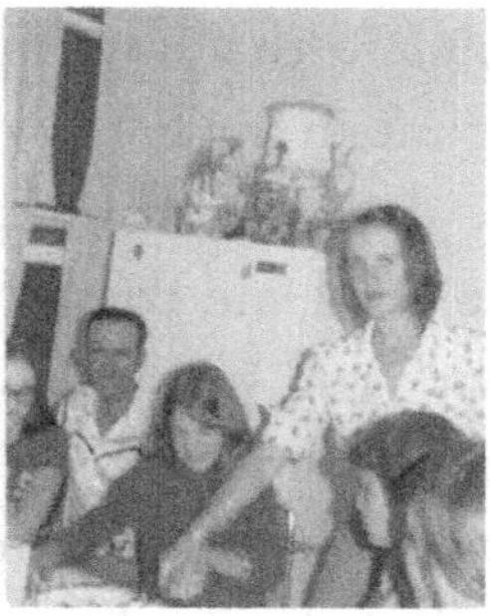

Chapter 25

The Trunk Never Left

"I no longer feared the darkness once I knew the Phoenix in me would rise from the ashes."
- W.C. Hannan.

I FOUND A LARGE APARTMENT on the top floor of a triplex on Park Avenue, in Uptown Montreal. It was an area I had never lived in before. Restaurants abounded, as did languages spoken on the streets; from Italian, Hebrew, Portuguese to ones I couldn't even guess their origins.

The important thing for me was that the apartment looked clean, had enough rooms for us and that the move took the kids away from the gangs and prostitution in Little Burgundy. I let the kids take charge of the apartment, painting the rooms whatever colour they chose. Part of me felt I was watching it happen from the outside, a spectator to it all.

The thought hit me that my input or help wasn't needed for the first time in my life.

My last baby, Baby Lorraine, wasn't so small anymore and didn't need me to watch her every step. The kids would fight as all kids do, but I was no longer required to kiss booboos or wipe tears.

I began babysitting the downstairs neighbour's kids a few days a week. It helped add to the money I was receiving from welfare, and I had not much else to do as I no longer worked at the diner or washed the businessmen's shirts.

Roger and I mostly saw each other on the weekends. He would pick me up, and we would go for drives or to stay in the basement of the brownstone. It was the only time I felt more like myself; on Overdale Street, where I knew everyone and where people cared that I was around. Roger made me feel wanted and loved. But then the weekend would end, and I would be back in a neighbourhood where I knew no one. In the house, everyone seemed to be too busy to spend time with me. My mini-boss had even started dating again. She was either out with her new beau, Peter, or at work. She did not come home often.

I felt alone.

With every passing day, my spirit began to dim. Even babysitting the neighbours' kids, which should have been enough to brighten my mood, started to feel like a chore. Going outside was no better; the neighbourhood was bustling with many nationalities, different smells, sounds and more to see; it was a lot to take in. Everything was foreign to me, and I felt like I didn't fit in.

I wasn't sleeping well, and I would often wake up feeling tired. When my feet would touch the floor, a voice of dread would creep into my head. The voice would say, "Why? Why get up? You don't have to do anything today." Then memories would flood my mind. Good and bad. The memories would bring tears to my eyes, and I would sit and not move. After a while, I would wipe my face and say to myself, "That's enough. Belle, go take care of everyone, and start them on their day." But when I was around my kids, I had no patience. I was so tired. I would hit them or yell at almost anything they would do wrong, then I would feel bad for overreacting. Even Buttons became nervous around me, but she never left my side; she still slept on the edge of my bed. Her presence didn't bring me much comfort. I felt I was letting her down like I was letting everyone down.

Sometimes in the middle of the day, I would find myself staring out the window at nothing, the tears would come, and I would curl up in a ball, alone and cry. I never questioned why this was happening. It felt like it was supposed to happen. I would be washing dishes, and a feeling of grief would come over me. The kids would ask, "Why are you crying, Mom?" I would tell them I heard a sad story that day and would rush off to the bathroom, closing the door behind me. Being around the kids or Roger was becoming hard. I knew they could sense something was wrong.

That's when I started to lie. I would say I was unwell so I could spend time alone in my room. Where are you, Belle? Who have you become, Belle? The darkest days were when I would try to figure out how to make it go away. I plotted for the swiftest and least gruesome way to end it all, so my children would not have to find me in a horrible scene of death.

Then I'd snap myself out of it. I was the only thing my kids had; I couldn't leave, and I'd lull myself to sleep. Unfortunately, the same thoughts would pop up again the next morning, continuously, each time bringing me further into the bad thoughts of leaving those I loved.

It must have been at least six months of this torment. Until one night, the darkness came over me, and I lost control. All of my fears, sadness, and memories took hold. The questions I had asked myself many times, "Where are you, Belle? Who is this? Why?" remained silent on my lips. I started to shake uncontrollably, pain and heat overtaking my body, yet I felt clammy and cold. I felt like I was dying, my heart beating hard in my chest.

I started to scream. My screaming could be heard throughout the house. Susan and Peter, who were watching TV, rushed into the bedroom where they found me. Susan tried to soothe me while Peter called for an ambulance. The paramedics checked my vitals; they were fine. But the paramedics could see that there was something wrong. I was still clammy, and my chest was heaving.

They brought me to the Montreal General Hospital. I was seen that night by a doctor, and he diagnosed me with severe depression. He said I had had a nervous breakdown.

The next day, I was released from the hospital and given a prescription for medication and appointments to see the doctor for follow-up visits. Roger brought me home. Susan had taken over my role as a parent; the house was clean, and she had made my bed. The kids all looked at me sadly, but none of them asked questions. I think Susan must have explained it to the younger kids. They never left me alone; outside of when I was in the washroom or asleep, one of the kids would always be near me.

At first, all I wanted to do was sleep. I was embarrassed to be around my children. I was embarrassed about not being Tuffy Belle, strong as an ox, now weak and vulnerable to the sadness in her head. As weeks passed and I took the medication and went to the doctor's visits, I slowly began to feel the darkness leaving.

I was raised to be a survivor. I had no choice, and down inside, I knew Mom would want me to figure out how to make it through. I had fought to make things work alone for too long. The trunk I had left in Overdale as a show of moving away from pain had only been a show. I broke because I was still carrying the weight of all of it by myself. I now knew I needed help to deal with my pain; all the losses life had dealt me.

Talking to the doctor helped me. The darkness had been in me since I lost Mom, I knew it would never fully disappear, but over the next year and a half that we lived on Park Avenue, I worked to let in the light. Some days were harder than others; some days, I still wanted to hide away in my bedroom. Those are the days I challenged myself to get up and clean, take care of the dogs and be around my kids. I never backed down from a fight and refused to back down from this one. I let go of my embarrassment of being weak. Once I did that, I began to find joy in spending time with my children; they still were a little too good to be their regular selves, but I could see they were starting to be more at ease. I was grateful for their care.

Belle is coming back.

Chapter 26
Mini-Boss

"Susan, you are a miracle of Grace." - L.H.

SUSAN STAYED HOME TO watch over me during my recovery. Her boyfriend Peter, wanting to be wherever his girlfriend was, quickly became a fixture in our apartment. Peter was a handsome young and responsible black man. Neither Susan nor Peter had reservations about dating someone outside of their race.

Susan, of course, could never be told no; she would do what she wanted anyway. Peter also seemed to know his own mind. From the first moment I met him, he let me know he had good intentions towards my daughter. It warmed my heart. I wanted my mini-boss to be happy with someone as strong as her.

By summer 1973, Susan and Peter had been dating for over a year. They sat me down in our living room and told me of their plans to get married. Peter had proposed the night before, and Susan had happily accepted. I was overjoyed.

Life was looking up. My depression had receded into something I could manage. The doctor had taken me off the medication, and I was hopeful for the future. My relationship with Roger was also going well. We had begun doing a lot more couple type activities, leaving the kids at home. Roger was the biggest country music lover; Johnny Cash was his idol. We began going to western bars. We loved to slow dance, and I just tucked right in the nook of his arm when he held me close. It was a part of my life that finally felt right. Roger knew I would never marry again or move in with him as long as I still had children at home, but we planned for a future when the kids were all grown. One thing I knew was that to continue healing, I needed to change where I lived. Uptown Montreal still felt foreign and unfriendly. I found a new apartment away from the bustle of downtown and uptown. It was in NDG, in the West End of Montreal, on Oxford Street, a beautiful duplex with a nice backyard. We would be living on the top floor. It felt like home—a place where I could feel proud to have guests over, and the kids could safely walk to the big park around the corner.

Because of the move, Carol, Jo-Ann and René Baby-La-La were transferred from Montreal High School to Monkland High. René Baby-La-La was always quiet, and he just blended in wherever he went; Carol and Jo-Ann had a more difficult time adjusting to the new school. They were in the last two years of high school, a hard time to settle in.

They would end up quitting soon after our move, preferring to find a job in an office or bank like their older sister. Susan now worked in the head office of the BMO bank; it showed the younger kids that they could succeed if they put their minds to it. Baby Lorraine, about to begin grade 5, was transferred to Herbert Symonds School and fit right in.

Daniel had stepped up since my breakdown. He would pay special attention to make sure the younger ones weren't hanging around the wrong people. Daniel had also gone back to school to become a certified auto mechanic, which would allow him to make more money working in the garage. He took the course seriously, trying to learn as much as he could. I can't remember a summer day when we lived on Oxford street, where the parking space in front didn't have a car in pieces with Daniel under it or that we didn't all gather in the living room in front of the TV for Hockey Night in Canada. Buttons even barked along with our cheers when the Montreal Canadians would score. I was happy again, it wasn't a perfect life, but it was perfect for me. You might say paradise found in NDG.

After living in the duplex for a year, the main floor apartment became available, and I jumped at the chance to move downstairs. As the tenant of the downstairs apartment, I'd have the use of the backyard. I loved it. I started to garden, something I hadn't done since I had lived with Grandma Nani. The kids even brought me seeds to plant.

My mini-boss Susan was busy planning for her wedding. The date had been set for spring 1975. The reception would be held at the duplex. I was so happy to have a nice home where I could host a party; it was far from the rat-infested rooming houses of before. As the day neared, I scrubbed the house spotless. Everyone took part in the preparations, decorating, cleaning and cooking.

I was given (my specialty) deviled eggs to make. Susan and the girls made sure to cook everything else and keep me out of the kitchen for the rest of the time (the nerve of them saying I could only do eggs!). The years of my not so stellar home cooking had left a mark on them.

On the day of the wedding, I was a bundle of nerves and yet beaming with happiness. As the church doors opened and the music started, there she was, a light to all, a beautiful young bride. Memories flooded my mind; her little hand in mine as she asked me so many years ago, "Mommy, are we moving again?" "Mom, can I have some milk too?" "Mommy, it will be okay Mom, cry Mommy, let it all out, I am here."

When she would come and lay quietly next to me, not saying a word because she knew I didn't need words, knowing I just needed to feel loved. There she stood, and my pride was overwhelming. She was God's angel, my lovely Susan. My little boss, my first baby of love, was all grown up. I cried tears of joy. My Susan had done well for herself. The ceremony was beautiful, and my smile didn't leave my face. Once the ceremony was over, I rushed back to the duplex to welcome the guests as they arrived.

The decorations were hung all over the house, and unlike receptions of people that rented fancy halls and ballrooms, this one had a special personal touch. There was an abundance of food and the drinks and laughter flowed all night. We had a great time with the guests. Auntie Sonya was older, but she showed up to the celebration with all the spunk of her younger self. Uncle Bob had long passed away, but Auntie always kept in touch with us. Doug and Loy refused to come; unfortunately, racism ingrained in our upbringing would not let go of them. I missed them not being there. Susan took their disapproval in stride. Not even the family's negativity towards Peter could damper her day.

My daughter's wedding, for me, was a true testament of love between two people. Susan was my daughter, and I believe my fire, my resolve, had been passed on to her. How could it not? Susan was my firstborn and had scraped and crawled her way along with me; when I dragged that trunk, she pushed it. Her devotion to those she loved was stronger than any I had ever encountered.

That night I danced. I danced with my heart full of joy for my children, new hope and love.

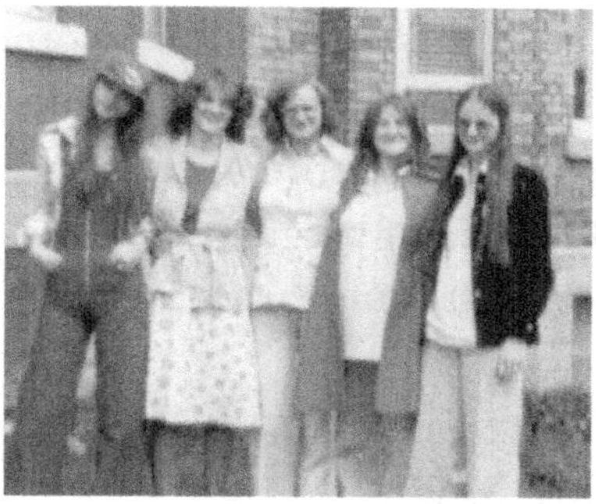

Chapter 27
Baby Kisses

"For you formed my inwards parts, you knitted me together in my mother's womb. I praise you, for I am fearfully and wonderfully made. Wonderful are your works; My soul knows it very well."- Psalm 139: 13-15

THE DECORATIONS WERE ALL taken down in the days following the wedding, and Susan packed up and moved out to the East End to begin her marriage with Peter. It was a bittersweet feeling to see her go.

I was proud and happy for her but also sad as I realized that life was changing. My home was emptier without her. Susan and Peter made it easier for me by visiting almost every day. Their constant visits made it that I could look forward to seeing my younger ones step out into the world. That ended up happening but not the way I expected.

Carol started to gain weight and wore looser clothes. She had also become very quiet. I noticed it, as did everyone else in the house. I knew something was up and worried about what it was. I went into her room and asked her if there was something wrong.

Carol told me, "I am pregnant."

I had suspected it but hearing it made me take a step back.

"By who?" I asked.

She wouldn't answer.

I can't explain what I was feeling; I just refused to accept another daughter pregnant at such a young age. When Susan had gotten pregnant, I had given her no choice; the baby needed to be raised in a good home. Susan, at 16, couldn't offer the child that.

With Carol, it was different. She was over 18 and had a job.

Do you want to keep the baby?"

She looked up at me and answered, "Yes."

I took a deep breath. It would be up to her, and I couldn't do much about it. Frustration overwhelmed me, and I blurted out, "You can't bring the baby here" then I left the room.

I was afraid. I was tired. I was not ready to help raise another child. I loved children, and yet I was letting my fear overtake my maternal instinct.

When Carol told the kids she was expecting, their emotions were mixed.

Daniel was upset, Susan supportive, and the rest didn't seem to know what to think. For the next few months, I would lie awake in my bed at night, tossing and turning. My guilt was consuming me. During the day, I was short with Carol. I tried to convince her to consider adoption and often would lose my patience with her.

Carol worked throughout the whole pregnancy. She paid for her food to ensure a healthy baby and stayed quiet while I would try to make her see the situation my way.

When her contractions started, Daniel drove us up to the hospital.

Carol delivered a baby boy. I left the room before the nurse cleaned him up. I did not want to see this baby. I could not handle that Carol was now a mother; I felt like I had failed my children by allowing her to get pregnant.

I gave Carol two weeks to find a new place to live. The baby remained at the hospital while Carol came home to figure out what to do. She went into her room and only came out to shower and eat. I had seen pain on my daughter's face many times before. But this time I had caused it. And yet, I refused to change my mind.

Susan and Peter came over and talked to Carol. Then they tried to speak to me; I said, "I don't want that baby here. Carol will have to move out if you bring him home," and yes, those were my words. As mean as it seemed. I had thought I would not see a teenage pregnancy again with my girls, and since I had, I was mad. And when you are mad, you say things you might later regret.

That same afternoon, the front door opened, and in walked Susan, Carol and Peter carrying a bundle. "I thought I told you not to bring him home!" As I said this, the baby was placed in my arms, and I didn't let go.

I kissed him, and kissed him and only then did I get a good look at him. He was beautiful, with big soulful brown eyes and light caramel skin, the first grandson that I would hold. Carol had named him Derek. A warm rush of pride hit me, and my heart grew larger to accept this much love for a child. I was undeniably a grandmother at the age of 43, and I loved it.

Derek and Carol stayed with us for two weeks until she found an apartment. I admit I failed her in her time of needing me.

I made her pregnancy harder than it needed to be. I live with this guilt. I was lucky that she still gave me a chance to get to know this beautiful baby.

I would babysit Derek when Carol went to work. Everyone loved Derek; he was the sweetest little boy. It was a fight between Jo-Ann and Baby Lorraine about who was going to get to hold him first. I stopped babysitting other kids, concentrating instead solely on my grandson.

On warm afternoons, I would install Derek's playpen outside, and all of Oxford Street would come over and visit us. Our dogs, Buttons and Bingo, would lay next to the playpen, always keeping a watchful eye on my new grandson.

I was able to stop babysitting other kids because Susan and Peter supported the family by ensuring we had enough food and helping me with the rent. I had indeed gained a son when Susan married Peter. And shortly, I will be gaining a new grandchild.

Susan was pregnant. Both she and Peter wanted Derek and his soon-to-be cousin to be close. As such, they spent the months before Susan gave birth, over at my duplex, getting to know their nephew.

My first granddaughter was born in 1976. Susan and Peter named her Lori (after Lorraine). She was the cutest little girl with big brown eyes and chubby cheeks. When Susan returned to work three months later, I took care of both Derek and Lori. I had my hands full, and I loved every minute of it.

By 1977, my little grandbabies were walking and talking. Derek was a curious toddler, getting into everything and a joy to be around. It was hard to believe I had once told Carol to put him up for adoption. I felt shame for my past actions, but Derek had opened my eyes to allowing love to win over everything. Taking care of him and Lori was becoming a highlight of my life. They also were showing me how quickly time passed and how things had changed. They were so tiny compared to my big kids. My children were now almost all adults outside of Baby Lorraine (and Baby Lorraine is now a baby only by name). They were spending a lot of time out of the house. Either they would be visiting at Susan's or Carol's or out with their boyfriends and girlfriends. I felt I wouldn't have all of them near for much longer, and I was right.

Daniel was now 23, and he came to me to tell me of his plans to marry. Jo-Ann, 20, followed her brother's news with her own. She was planning to get married to her beau Stephen, a kind-hearted young man she had been dating for over a year. The kicker was that they both wanted to have their weddings in the same month! They both also wanted the receptions to be held at the duplex! We ran around like crazy to organize the two receptions. Once again, the food would be all homemade, and we rehung the decorations we had used for Susan's wedding. The only hiccup turned out to be due to their success. The guests were enjoying themselves so much they drank all the alcohol at Jo-Ann's wedding! Susan and Peter had to get some more liquor, and the party continued. At both weddings, I danced and danced. Roger was twirling me around as we celebrated life and family. I felt so happy, so complete with my children, grandchildren, and boyfriend. I wanted to yell out loud, "I am Belle, and I am so happy!"

What a whirlwind life had become.

Chapter 28
Cute As A Button

"Every dog is a lion at home." - Henry George Bohn.

MY DOGS, BUTTONS AND BINGO, had become a big part of my life; they provided me with security and joy. Susan and Peter added to that by bringing me a Saint Bernard dog named Supe. She was gorgeous, with big droopy eyes and floppy ears. I fell for her instantly.

Susan and Peter wanted us to breed her to make money. The deal was that I would house and take care of her, and they would find the buyers for her puppies when the time came. I agreed. I had done many odd jobs in my life, from night watchman to washerwoman, but never had I had a job that promised such adorable trouble.

The duplex basement was soon full of our three dogs and Supe's litter of eight puppies. It was hard to go downstairs without tripping over an excited pup. Supe wasn't maternal at all. Heck! When she gave birth, we even had to help her push them out; she just laid there like a fat lump on a log. She also refused to feed them. The kids and I had to bottle feed all eight pups. It was tiresome but sweet. At times I wondered if I had taken on more than I had bargained for; eight mouths to feed every couple of hours drained me more than babysitting my two grandbabies. They managed to sell the pups as soon as they were weaned off milk. We shared the money and concluded that we wouldn't breed her again.

Supe just wasn't mommy material. But the experience had made us all fall in love with the Saint Bernard breed of dogs, so much so that Susan and Peter decided to buy another one, a beautiful Saint Bernard show dog named Jake.

Since they were still living in an apartment, they kept him at my house. To be fair, after having lived with eight puppies, one more dog didn't bother me. I had begun to see the dogs as part of my family. They even misbehaved like some of my children. Jake was a perfect example of that. He was a giant blob who would occasionally sneak out. Usually, someone from the neighbourhood would spot him and bring him home. It wasn't hard to bring him back; he was incredibly friendly with everyone and would dutifully follow them. He seemed perfectly happy, and then he would try to slip away again.

When Peter and Susan purchased their home, they left me Supe but took Jake with them. I couldn't blame them; Jake was a big bundle of troublesome love. The kids took Jake leaving as a sign to bring me more animals ranging from dogs to canaries, and I accepted them all.

I made sure our house was always clean, even with all the pets. It kept me busy in the evening. I only had René Baby-La-La and Baby Lorraine living at the duplex. Everyone else would come to visit daily, but it would be just the three of us as the night neared. I think René Baby-La-La was starting to feel like he was too old to be still living at home. A house full of pets and a younger teenage sister didn't appeal to him. Soon after Susan had purchased her house, he got a job at the

Eaton's department store in downtown Montreal and moved closer to his job.

The duplex was now quiet and felt too big and empty. Susan stopped working when she became pregnant with her second child, Peter Christopher, and kept Lori with her. Carol was always at Susan's house with Derek, so I didn't babysit him anymore either. What a switch from a full home to a now near-empty one. Even Daniel came around less as his wife had just given birth to a baby boy. They had named him René after his father. Daniel was busy working to provide for his son. He was now an aerial mechanic and soon would be working as an engineer. It didn't leave a lot of time to visit his mother. Nor to be a good husband, as he and his wife divorced shortly after Peter Christopher's third month.

Baby Lorraine and I moved, leaving our beautiful duplex in exchange for a smaller two-bedroom apartment. The apartment was on Côte Saint-Luc street, right beside a synagogue, higher up from Oxford. It was still located close enough that Baby Lorraine would be able to continue to attend Monkland High School. With my days empty, I decided to get a job working with children. I became a nanny to two kids named Dylan and Petra. They called me Auntie Belle. It felt good to be useful again. Roger had encouraged me to take the job. He knew how important it was for me to be around children.

Baby Lorraine was about to be 16 and always out and about with friends. She had matured differently than my other daughters. Baby Lorraine was taller but also seemed to be less interested in boys than my other girls. She was my tomboy. She loved to play football and roughhouse with our dogs. Her love for our dogs made what was to come very hard on our relationship.

Buttons had been the last gift from my husband, René, before he died in 1967. It was now 1978, and her age was beginning to show; she was not doing well. I took her to the veterinarian and was told she was in pain. I had to put Buttons down. I felt more than sadness for a beloved pet; It was also a final goodbye to the life I used to live. I loved that dog. I could still remember saying, "René, I can't afford another mouth to feed and not a half-crippled dog."

It was a trying day. I shed a lot of tears. When Baby Lorraine got home from school, I had to tell her, and she said, "Mom, why did you kill my dog, the one thing I had left from my father!" It broke my heart. I hoped that Baby Lorraine would soon realize I hadn't done it to hurt her.

She was distant for months after Buttons died. It was a lonely time for me. I wanted my Baby Lorraine back; she only had a few years of high school left, and then she might leave. I wanted the next few years to be happy. By the end of November, she started talking with me.

The year 1978 was coming to a close, and although our relationship had somewhat improved, I still felt she was not her usual self. I soon found out why.

It was early in the evening when there was a knock at the door. When I went to open it, Baby Lorraine and a handsome, neatly-dressed, dark-skinned young man were standing in the doorway. "Hello Mrs. Lessard, my name is Darrell."

Baby Lorraine's eyes were popping out; she looked nervous and didn't say a word. "Come in, Darrell. Lorraine, why are you just standing there? Invite your guest in." That was when I realized my tomboy, my Baby Lorraine, had been distant for more reasons than I knew. She had a beau.

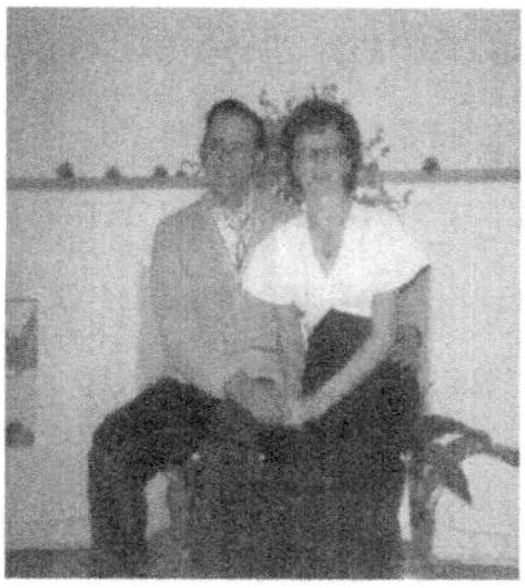

Chapter 29
My Cowboy

"Sing your death song and die like a hero
Going home." - Chief Tecumseh

AS 1979 ROLLED IN, Baby Lorraine and Darrell spent quite a lot of time together. Now that my youngest was happy and settled, she didn't mind if I wasn't around as much.

I started to spend more nights with my sweetheart Roger. For years, Baby Lorraine had made me feel guilty when I would leave for the night. It wasn't because she didn't like Roger, but because I was all she had outside of her siblings.

I was happy that she was in a good relationship, and I could now give Roger more attention.

For so many years, Roger had stood by me; he had been okay with my house rules and my need to raise my children as I saw fit. I had lucked out when he picked me up at that diner.

It was nice to now be able to have our relationship become the central part of our lives. We continued to go to western bars, drives, and all our other activities, but the nights we cuddled in bed stood out for me as our most memorable time together. Roger held me tight and made me feel safe.

By mid-summer, though, he had begun to worry me. My strong silent man was complaining quite often of fatigue. This was not like him. He had never complained about anything before. I begged him, "Roger, you have to go see a doctor." Roger was stubborn. He refused to go to a white man's doctor; being of Indian descent, he didn't believe in medical doctors. Roger had always looked fit. He had a few bad habits like smoking rolled cigarettes from the Indian reserve and his appetite for steak and potatoes. But I had always seen those as his 'man habits.'

One hot and humid summer night in 1979, the phone rang after I had already gotten into bed. I was alone in the apartment and ran to answer it; our phone was in the living room. I picked it up on its fourth ring, and all I could hear was gasping on the line, and then Roger's voice hoarse (as if in pain) uttered, "Belle...Belle...help!"

The phone went dead. I quickly called an ambulance and then Jo-Ann. I was crying. I told her that something had happened to Roger, and to please get me. Jo-Ann and Stephen lived over on Somerled Avenue, only a few blocks from my apartment. Stephen called Daniel to meet us at Roger's as Jo-Ann got dressed. They rushed over to pick me up. My apartment was a

10-minute drive from Overdale. As we pulled up, the police and the ambulance were already there. The police let me enter the apartment. The paramedics were in his living room. As I entered, they moved, and I saw him slumped in his chair. I was too late; Roger had died of a massive heart attack. I went to him, fell to my knees and held his hand, it was still warm, and I caressed his hair. Daniel came to me, and I cried in his arms. Jo-Ann was sobbing on Stephen's shoulders. At that moment, I hated life, and I hated Overdale. I muttered, "No good, this Overdale never no good. It has taken my sweetheart," and then I yelled, "Fuck you, Overdale!" and Daniel held me tighter.

I needed someone or something to blame. I was in shock at losing another lover to a heart attack. I couldn't believe it. My big Cowboy, my sweetheart, came into my life when I needed him the most, and never asked us for anything, only gave of himself, and loved the children. A man who had endured rejection and abuse in his childhood yet had not let that bitter him—my silent warrior. Just as the children had almost all settled and we were about to be able to move in together, he was no longer here. My tears stopped, and I felt empty inside.

"I am alone again." I went and sat on the hard cement window ledge of the brownstone for what seemed like hours and yet could have been minutes as I waited for the coroner to arrive. Time no longer mattered.

The tears flowed again once I was back home, in my bed. This time my confidante was not there to console me, nor were my warrior's arms there to hold me. The days following Roger's death were a haze as the kids helped me plan his funeral. All of them were there for me.

The morning of the funeral, I woke to the sound of Jewish men singing hymns in the Synagogue next door. I had never paid attention to these hymns, but today they comforted me. I found myself humming Amazing Grace; it's one of my favourite hymns, and it felt right and just as a tribute to a man who had discovered his amazing grace. I dressed in a black pantsuit and left my hair loose. Roger had often said he liked me in pantsuits and dresses because he liked how my legs looked. I wanted to look pretty for him one last time, even though I felt lost.

My children and I were the only ones in attendance at the funeral. Roger had no family he spoke to, just us. He was always welcome on the reserve in Kahnawake but would never stay. None of them came to pay their respects, nor did the people at his job.

He should have had the whole of Montreal there. He was special. He made his way from the hardest of beginnings. Indians had a hard time finding work and were thought of as drunks and unreliable. Being homeless as a teenager in Montreal, he lived with the stigma of being an Indian and had to prove many times he was a hard-working man and did not believe in drinking. He never let what people thought deter him from getting what he wanted.

As the pastor began his sermon, my mind drifted back to the first time I had seen him; his dark looks and tall, strong frame had caught my eye right away. He had those big chains and, of course, the turquoise rings that many Indians wore. He was so handsome.

What should I do now?

Roger has been part of our family. He supported me in all my struggles and gave me all he could. Roger loved my kids unconditionally.

He accepted them as individuals and didn't overstep and try to parent them. In all our years together, there was only one time he yelled at my kids, which was for a good reason. René Baby-La-La and Jo-Ann had always been up to some mischief when they were younger. They would spend most of their childhood summers out and coming home when the streetlights came on; that was my rule. On one of their excursions, they went into an old, abandoned building. I had forbidden them to go in there because of how dangerous it was. Kids being kids, they hadn't listened. They went in and found old bones, which they brought back home and tried piecing together in the alleyway. Roger caught them and yelled up a storm, and they ran inside. He told me about it. He apologized for yelling at my kids but said how he couldn't stand by and let them play with bones that had been laid to rest. He had been raised with traditional beliefs that desecrating an old burial ground would disturb spirits and cause trouble. He was always looking out for my family. Even after he yelled at her, Jo-Ann didn't take it badly. She took him as the father figure she never had.

As the ceremony came to a close, and we were walking back, I kept thinking of how my children and I had benefited from having him in our lives. His support and love had been given so freely and fully, I had taken for granted that it would always be present. Once in a lifetime, you will find a connection built on mutual respect and not a one-sided romance. I love René forever, but he never respected me the way Roger did. Roger thought the world of me, and all he wanted in return was to be loved and respected. I did, and forever he would have a piece of my heart.

Chapter 30
Naughty Belle

"When you are not fed love on a silver spoon, you learn to lick it off knives." -Lauren Eden

A FEW MONTHS AFTER Roger's death, Jo-Ann and Stephen asked if Baby Lorraine and I would like to co-rent a duplex.

It would help us both out as far as expenses go and help them save up to purchase a house in the future. I happily accepted. The place we rented was on Isabella Avenue, a few blocks from the apartment. I was upstairs with Baby Lorraine, and Jo-Ann was downstairs. My position as a nanny was not full time, and I was home a lot. Everyone else, including Baby Lorraine, worked and stayed out and busy.

I could see Baby Lorraine's attention was fading from school. She spent all of her free time with her beau Darrell or working her part-time job. Right after her 18th birthday, Baby Lorraine told me she would not be returning to school. She was dropping out and moving in with Darrell.

My greatest fear was that she would end up like me. Maybe she would not have as many kids, but they were starting out with nothing, like René and I had. I wanted better for her, and I didn't mince my words or keep my voice down as I tried to get through to her. My yelling, my anger, even my pleas to not leave, didn't stop her. All my children were stubborn. I think they got it from me, but it still didn't make me appreciate that trait in them. How could they not see that all I wished was for them to succeed and for our family to be close?

My whole life, I wanted to love and be loved and now I had no one, not a child in my home, not a lover in my bed. I missed being held at night. I missed Roger. It's scary how someone can be part of your life for so long and yet disappear from it so quickly. I had lost many I cared for; Roger was now part of that awful list. One of the things that I had thought would make it easier with Roger was that I had never lived with him.

When I would wake up from bed, I didn't expect to see him beside me, nor to see him facing me at supper. I had told myself I would be alright; I was Tuffy Belle. Tuffy Belle rolled with the punches and dealt with the losses. For a whole year, I had tried to pretend my heart wasn't broken, that I wasn't lonely and that I had moved on by returning to tending the kids under my care and providing for Baby Lorraine and myself.

But now, in the empty upstairs duplex, I couldn't pretend any longer. I was lonely. I was 48 years old, single and I felt starved for affection.

Every day I would take the bus to go to my job. One day as I was getting on the bus to go home, I tripped over a step, and a young man steadied me. I looked up to thank him and found myself staring up at the thickest coke bottle rimmed glasses that I have ever seen. He was staring back into my eyes. I looked away and mumbled a thank you. He wasn't incredibly handsome, and was of average height and build, but for some odd reason, when our eyes had connected, it had caused a reaction inside me. He smiled, followed me to my seat and introduced himself. His name was Gerry. We talked non-stop the whole 20-minute ride, and when I got off the bus, he got off with me. Gerry was flirting and I was flirting back; it was like a little devil was whispering into my ear. I know I should wish him a good day and leave, but I didn't want the conversation to end. I felt a rush of daring, something like when I was a young teenager, a little naughty. I found myself asking him if he had time to go for coffee. For the rest of the afternoon, we sat and talked. I told him some stories about my life, and he just listened as if he cared. It felt good to have male attention. Before he left, I gave him my number. He called me a few days later to meet up again. It wasn't long before I took a foolish leap and found myself in bed with him. I have never been shy to say that I enjoy sex. I have six kids, and it was not the baby stork who dropped them off!

Gerry was different from all the other men I had dated. He was almost 16 years younger than me, and he did drugs. I had never been with someone who smoked weed. There was a spirit of abandonment when we were together; no serious conversations or responsibilities, just fun and wantonness. He always had a wild story to tell, and he made me feel like a young woman.

Who was I becoming? I didn't know, but I did know I liked it. I started to invite him over to the duplex. He would meet me at the bus stop as I got off, and he and I would spend the afternoons enjoying each other. He would leave before Jo-Ann and Stephen returned from work. On the third time over, I tried weed at his urging. I coughed at the first toke of the joint, and I felt silly and giggled.

One afternoon I hadn't noticed the time passing, and Jo-Ann and Stephen walked into my apartment while Gerry and I were sharing a joint. Gerry had his feet up on the coffee table, and Jo-Ann could not have been more shocked. "Hello Mom, are you ok? Who are you?" she asked Gerry. I quickly cleaned up and rushed Gerry out. "Jo-Ann, I am a full-grown woman, and I am your mother, and if I want company, I will have company. It is my fucking business!"

Jo-Ann stormed downstairs with Stephen behind her and slammed the door. She came and tried to reason with me and to tell me that Gerry was not a person I should have in my life. I refused to listen; I was not about to stop seeing Gerry.

It was a rough six months.

Jo-Ann and I were always arguing. She would yell, "Mom, I can't take the smell of weed all the time," and I would shrug my shoulders and tell her to fuck off. Before dating Gerry, I used to curse only when I was upset.

Now I sounded like a drunken sailor, with every other word being a curse word. Jo-Ann started to stay away.

Gerry would come and go and never confide in me where he spent his time or about anything really! Our relationship wasn't stable or deep. I started to feel like it had been a silly indulgence and a thoughtless one. My guilt was mounting about the distance it had created with my daughter. I finally broke off with Gerry when

Jo-Ann and Stephen announced she was pregnant. But the damage was done.

Jo-Ann, angry and hurt, broke the lease, and we went our separate ways. As she packed her things, Jo-Ann expressed her disappointment in me and mentioned many of her things were stolen by Gerry. I didn't believe her at the time. I didn't believe I wouldn't have seen him steal or that I would have been with a crook, but I felt awful for the hurt that I had caused her. Never had I treated one of my children with such disrespect. I packed my things and moved into a small apartment.

This time I only had my regrets accompanying me.

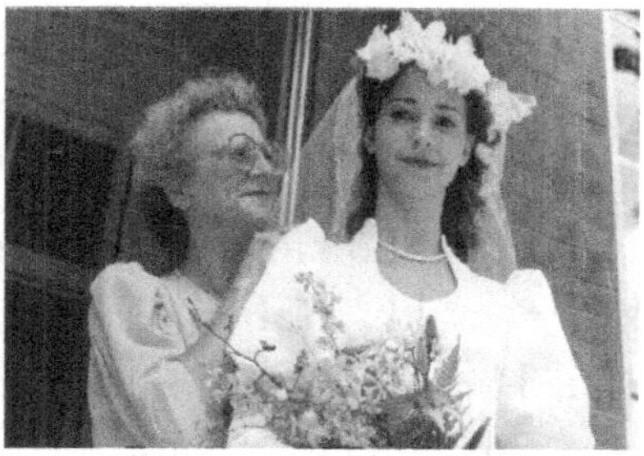

Chapter 31
Fooled

"I can enjoy anywhere and I can leave it. Life is about moving on." - Warris Dirie.

I WANT TO SAY THAT was the end of my fling with Gerry, but it would be a lie. I did stop talking to him for many months, and during that time, my Jo-Ann had her beautiful baby, a daughter they named Natasha.

For the next bit of time, I tried very hard to smooth the bumps that the last year had caused in my relationships with Jo-Ann and Baby Lorraine. And for a while, being a mother and grandmother was enough.

Then, Gerry called me. At first, it was just a hello and some conversation. It was nice, and it felt good to feel like I was missed.

A few weeks passed, and then he called again, this time to go out for a coffee.

I had a hard time refusing someone I had been with in the past.

We met up and did a bit more than talk. As I left, I told myself it was just a stolen moment, a little day thrill that wouldn't happen again. And it wouldn't for a while, and then he'd come around, and it would happen again. I didn't think it would go further than the casual flirtation that it had become.

I was adamant that I didn't want him in my house. But our few moments together kept me from feeling lonely. I had just had both my sons Daniel and René Baby-La-La move away to Vancouver. As all my babies had left me to become their own people, it felt good to feel like someone wanted to be with me.

My last baby, Baby Lorraine, came over with Darrell in early 1984 to announce they were getting married in July. She asked me to make her veil and the ring cushion. I felt honoured and set off right away on my task. Memories of "Mommy, Mommy, teach me French," "Mommy, hold my hand and don't go," floating in my head with every stitch I made in the fabric. I could still feel her little hand in mine. How was she getting married already? Tears welled in my eyes.

On the day of the wedding, there was not a dry eye in the church. Ranee, Darrell's mother, had sewn Baby Lorraine's dress. She looked breathtaking in it as she walked down the aisle.

The reception was held at a venue, which meant no deviled eggs to prepare or decorations to hang. The guests all gathered in the hall and danced for hours. It was beautiful to see; we were a mixture of black, white and everything in between, all connected, all family, dancing and happy.

I would never have brought Gerry to the wedding, but as I saw all of my kids content with their significant others, I felt a tingle of regret for being by myself. Did I make a mistake by keeping Gerry at arm's length?

Shortly after the wedding, I decided to let him fully back into my life. He moved in with me. I had rules for him. He had to get a job and not smoke weed in the house. I also told him I was not going to smoke weed. Gerry said yes to all of it.

He made me feel safe as we would spend a lot of time together. He smoked outside of the apartment and then would come inside, where we would spend all our evenings laughing and making love. It wasn't all roses. Gerry often got fired from jobs, and those he would get were not very high paying. His weed habit was quite expensive to maintain, and add it to buying food for two people; we were often short on cash.

The old practice of moving into different cheaper apartments reared its ugly head. I got a new job working as a mother's helper to ensure we could pay rent, and soon Gerry found a better paying job, working at an auction house.

My children were not happy about my relationship, but it was my life. I deserved to be with someone. The wedding had shown me they were all leading their own lives. Didn't I deserve a partner as well?

I tried to lessen the impact of going back to him by being more present for Jo-Ann, the one I had hurt the most the first time I had been with Gerry. Jo-Ann was pregnant with her second child. As the year continued, my children added to the count of my expected grandchildren. Daniel had remarried in Vancouver, where his new wife was pregnant, and Baby Lorraine was expecting her first baby. They gave birth a few weeks apart. Baby Lorraine's son Darrell Junior had some health issues and stayed in the hospital for a long time. Jo-Ann had given birth to a healthy son, Cory. I gave Baby Lorraine her space while I helped tend to Jo-Ann's two kids. Unfortunately, the distance made it that I wouldn't get to see my grandson Oliver, Daniel's son, for a long time. I tried hard to balance my relationship with Gerry and to be there for every one of my kids. But having six kids makes for many grandkids, and I always felt like I wasn't giving someone enough attention.

I knew I hadn't been there enough for Susan over the last few years. She was having difficulty in her marriage with Peter. I didn't realize how serious the trouble was until they separated and divorced in 1987. We all loved Peter and saw him as a member of our family. It was a hard time, and there were many conflicts as the kids tried to decide where their allegiance stood, Susan or Peter. Oddly, the divorce drama made it so that the kids stopped pestering me about my relationship with Gerry.

The moment the attention wasn't on how we were doing seemed to be the moment where everything crumbled. Gerry was working late a lot. I had noticed but had so much on my plate that I was happy he kept himself busy. We did have a few arguments, but nothing out of the ordinary.

Until the day in 1988, over breakfast, he announced, "I am leaving. I have someone else, and she is pregnant." My jaw went slack, and my mouth dropped open. I was shocked by the news, and I left the room. There was nothing left for me to say to this man.

As I sat on my bed, the first thing that came into my mind was, "Belle, here you go again, but at least he didn't die of a heart attack!"

After Gerry moved out, I began to realize how many things were missing. Over the years, my children had given me items that I cherished—gone, gone, gone. He had stolen them all!

Jo-Ann had told me many years ago he was a thief. Why hadn't I believed her? I can't say I had been blinded by love; this man had never held a piece of my heart. I should have done better and accepted the truth.

I didn't cry. I was so mad at myself. I went to the owner of the apartment building and told him I was moving out. I needed to get away from anything that reminded me of my foolishness and Gerry. My daughters were now all residing on the South Shore, in the town of Chambly. I decided to get an apartment over there and out of Montreal. I saw moving there as a fresh new start. As I packed my things, I kept repeating, "Belle, you'll get it right one day."

Chapter 32
Belle Is Getting Married

"Love has no age, no limit; and no death."
- John Galsworthy.

THE ONE MESSAGE I'VE tried to get through to my kids is that family comes first and you must always love and protect each other.

No one on this earth can share what you as my children share, my blood, strength, and the force that kept us together through thick and very thin. In the next few years, our family grew and grew, and with it, the love and the bond we shared. Carol had a second son, Alex and Jo-Ann, had another child, Crystal, and Baby Lorraine had her second child, Kyell. Daniel outdid them all by having another three kids and getting married for the third time! My family had changed from baby boots to miniskirts to marriage and divorce. As it changed, the importance of trying to keep family first mattered more than ever.

Luckily my move to Chambly had been timely. I was able to spend more time with my grandkids, showing them that they were loved. They were my world.

The only time I wasn't with them was when I'd babysit a few neighbourhood kids. The rest of the time I was the best grandma I could be. I went to all of my grandkids (the ones who lived in Quebec) sporting events.

By 1994, I was 62 years old, and I was the proudest and loudest seasoned fan and grandmother at the rink and the gym. It was exciting to watch them play and to attend their games and competitions.

At one of the hockey games, I met another grandparent who cheered his grandkids on as much as I did. I met my match; his name was Gerald Patrick O'Brien. I told him I'd call him Patrick. We hit it off immediately.

The next game, he was already sitting on the bleachers when I got there. I joined him, and we spent the first half of the game cheering on our grandsons and boasting about how great they were. At the intermission, he asked if I wanted to get some hot chocolate. As we got back to our seats and the next period started, we once again went back to cheering our grandsons on. Both of us were so excited that we jumped up when one of our grandsons scored, which caused us to knock over our drinks. It didn't matter; we were too happy to care. Patrick was fun to be with, and he just brought out the giggly girl I had buried a long time ago. He didn't have much hair, and he wasn't tall, but his eyes were a shining Irish blue, and his smile was contagious; I couldn't help but smile back. Soon I found out he was also a great kisser!

We became a cute "golden years" couple. Patrick would pick me up to go to the hockey games, and he introduced me to his Legion buddies.

He was a veteran and spent a lot of his time at the Legion, where he was an active member. We would go there to reminisce about our youth, and to see friends and dance. He was terrific on the dance floor. After dating for over a year and a half, Patrick asked me to be his wife. It felt so right to say yes. Patrick was a man who valued family as much as I did, and more than that, he made me feel happy in the morning as I got up and content at night when I would lay my head down to sleep.

I was excited to tell my kids about my plans to wed. They were all happy for me except for Baby Lorraine. She gave me such a fight, just like when she was a little girl, and I had plans to go out with Roger. For the first time in my life, I didn't try to entertain my youngest daughter's cries.

I told Baby Lorraine, "Stop it. Mommy deserves happiness at this time in my life. Get over it." She sulked many times after when we were together. But as the wedding neared, she began to understand that her pouting wasn't going to change my mind and that Patrick was right for me.

I made sure to involve my daughters in planning my wedding day. Patrick and I also wanted our wedding to include our grandchildren as much as possible. They would all have roles to play on our special day, and be dressed up in beautiful matching outfits, the boys in black and white with bow ties and the girls in long black and white dresses. I loved planning and shopping with my daughters. I had spent so many years scrimping and only purchasing clothes from the Salvation Army; as I shopped for my wedding dress, I realized how much my life had changed. For once, shopping wasn't about finding the cheapest dress out of necessity. It was about the pleasure of being with my girls and finding the perfect outfit for the upcoming event. A rush of warmth and a sense of comfort ran through me. I stopped mid-sentence at the dress shop. I sat, and I cried.

"Mom, what is wrong?" Jo-Ann asked.

I caught my breath and said, "She is here."

"Who is here?"

"My mom is here. I can feel her presence and hear her singing and see her dancing. She wants me to know this is my turn to feel happiness, and she is here in my heart, and she is happy for me. I love all of you." I smiled and then said, "This will be the best wedding ever."

I bought a beautiful two-piece powder pink long dress. I decided that I'd add a beautiful white peony in my hair, which was Mom's favourite flower.

I left the dress shop that day, bubbling over in happiness.

The ceremony would be held at St. Stephen Church in Chambly, and of course, the reception at the Legion. The day before the wedding, the whole wedding party had gone to decorate the Legion. We put up thousands of mini lights and big white bows tied with pink ribbons. The tables' centerpieces were lanterns and filled with small miniature lights. Giant balloons were everywhere. And when it was all done, we turned on all the lights, and it looked like a fairy tale, only I would make sure I did not wear glass slippers. I wanted to ensure that this fairy tale night I had planned would last.

The morning of the wedding, I got dressed with my daughters at Peter's house. Once all dressed up, the family gathered to take pictures before heading out to the church. A limousine came to pick me up. It arrived late to the church, maybe a little later than it should, but traditionally all brides show up a bit late, don't they?

Derek, my oldest grandson, was waiting to help me out of the car. He took my hand from the limousine and held it as we made our way into the church and down the aisle. All of the grandkids followed behind us. Patrick and I wanted all of them to give me away. In his black suit and white shirt, Patrick looked so handsome as he stood by the altar. I smiled. We were lucky to have one another and even luckier to be surrounded by those we loved; the service was attended by our entire family, my side and Patrick's. René Baby-La-La and Daniel had flown in from Vancouver, and Doug made it with his family and Loy with hers. It felt good that the people I held dear had come to celebrate and support my marriage to Patrick. The reception was a party that would have made Aunt Sonya proud. We danced and danced and laughed until our bellies hurt. I didn't stop smiling and kissing my new husband the whole night.

Belle was finally ready to live. I had been everything everyone needed, everyone wanted, no matter how much it cost me, and now I was finally putting my happiness first. I know René would have approved, and Roger would have cheered.

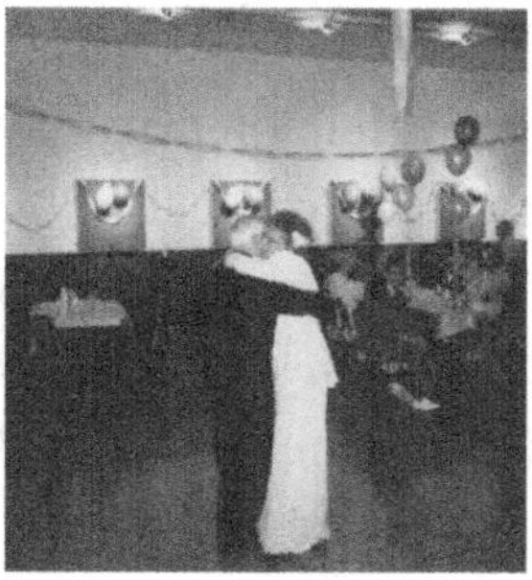

Chapter 33
Daffodils

"Your joy can fill you only as deeply as your sorrow has carved you." - Khalil Gibran.

AFTER THE WEDDING, PATRICK gave his house to his children. He wanted us to have something new, something that would be our own.

We purchased a trailer home. It was perfect, big enough for us two, and waiting for us to put our mark on it. I was over the moon; I was a homeowner! I was so proud. I never imagined owning a home. It was like I had become a sixty-something Cinderella! The prince of my dreams and now our place, our palace.

Patrick and I worked hard on the trailer to make it ours. We spent full afternoons at the garden centers picking the perfect flowers for our front yard and flower boxes. The flowers were not just for any old garden; they were for my garden. Belle's garden. I chose beautiful daffodils and peonies to plant in the front yard and filled my window boxes with pretty daisies. Every purchase and every improvement felt special. Patrick and I wanted the inside of our home to feel as welcoming as the outside was becoming. We painted and decorated the house with bright colours. We also made sure to have cut flowers in our home. It felt fresh, clean and absolutely perfect.

In the evenings, Patrick would rock in his chair and smile as I fussed over the littlest details in our home. Patrick had always owned his home. He marvelled at how happy and magical I found our place to be. I had to keep pinching myself and telling myself, "Yes, Belle. It is real. You have found your Eden."

Sometimes when I would visit my daughters, they would ask me to stay over for the night, something I had always jumped at the chance to do. I would grin and say, "Sorry, I can't. I have to go home." We had five beautiful years like this — years that seemed to pass in the blink of an eye.

In 2000, my forever after started to slip from my fingers. Patrick was not feeling well; he had stomach pain, continuous heartburn, and he'd begun to pass blood when he'd go to the washroom. We made a doctor's appointment. The doctor was concerned and ordered tests. After many tests, the doctor called us to come in for another appointment. As we sat in the doctor's office, the doctor told Patrick, "I'm sorry, Mr. O'Brien, but you have stage 4 stomach cancer. It is inoperable. You have six months to live."

We asked the doctor if there were any options, and he very sadly stated, "You can try chemotherapy, but it is uncomfortable and will only prolong your suffering Mr. O'Brien."

The drive home was silent. I dreaded getting home. It was a place of magical joy. We had had such a short time to indulge in it. Our home now seemed to scream out at me that all joy would soon disappear.

Patrick went to our room and asked to be alone for a bit, and I was relieved because I needed time to think. I felt raw with grief; Why me? Why did I have to lose everyone I loved? And how would I ever let this man go? I loved him!

I put on my coat and went out for a short walk around the trailer park. While the tears were falling down my cheeks, I thought about how every moment in my life was brief, good or bad. I could not take the bad moments back or stop the clock. I wanted too badly, but it was not about me or my pain. It was about Patrick. The man who had only brought happiness to my life. He needed me strong now more than ever. I had to make it that he felt love and joy around him. And with that thought, I decided to do everything I could to make the ending of his story beautiful and full of love.

I wiped my tears and entered our palace, embracing the love that lived there.

Patrick had fallen asleep, so I left him to rest, and I began my phone calls. One by one, I called my family, and I told them the news. I explained how important it was that these next months be the happiest ones we could offer Patrick.

I specifically told each of them, "Please, don't cry around Patrick, smile and give him the same hugs you always do. Patrick needs us to show him how happy we are to be with him, not because he's dying, but because he's the man we love."

When he woke up a little later on in the evening, Patrick and I talked well into the night. We spoke of our meeting for the first time, of silly Baby Lorraine shouting at us against our marriage plans, and the love of our grandchildren. We eventually fell asleep in each other's arms.

The next day we did not talk about cancer. Like any other day, we planned our activities, picked some fresh flowers, and set off to visit our close friend who just had a baby. Patrick was the type of man who made friends quickly, no matter their age.

This friend had been his boss, a pizza shop owner, as Patrick had delivered pizzas for him as his retirement gig. We were both excited to meet this new tiny baby. We knew he would warm our hearts.

As the weeks passed, our families did as I requested, and we shared good times with them. Some other days were filled with visits from friends. But soon, a lot of our time was spent at home. Patrick was feeling tired and rundown.

The disease was taking him rapidly, and he continued to lose a lot of weight. I tried to keep up the upbeat demeanour, but it was trying. Sometimes I would sneak a moment when Patrick took naps, and I would let it all out. I did it mostly in the shower where no one could hear me, and I could let the grief wash over me. The glass slippers were off; those moments did not feel part of a fairy tale.

My children were always voicing their concern for my health, but I knew my health wasn't important right now. Only Patrick mattered. This was the first time I had to watch someone I love slip away. I don't know which was worse, watching this horrible disease as it slowly robbed me of him or receiving a phone call in the night with no time to say goodbye. In the end, the pain of loss was the same.

As Christmas approached, I kept changing my mind on how to make it memorable for Patrick. I wanted to have our family over, but our home was too small, and it would be too much for us to plan a dinner at our house. My kids understood and decided they would host us for Christmas dinner.

Peter, my ex-son-in-law, offered his home for the party. It was large and could hold our whole family, Patrick's family and a few special guests.

The children prepared a tribute to him during the evening. They had rehearsed a song and sang it for Patrick. It was beautiful, and by the end of it, we were all in tears.

As 2001 moved in, it brought harder days. Patrick had become too weak to stay in our home. He was transferred to the hospital.

He was there for a full month—a month of visits with dear ones that wanted to say goodbye. Late at night, when everyone was gone and visiting hours were over, I would climb up next to him and hum a song, hoping to soothe both of us.

I would fall asleep with him in his hospital bed and dream of what could have been.

One morning when I woke up, he was gone. His hand was cold in mine, but where I had laid my head on his chest, his heart was warm. I cried and cried.

That spring, the daffodils were not bright and cheerful. Even my home seemed dark and dreary. Everywhere I looked, I felt something was missing. Patrick was missing. Without him, everything felt wrong. I began to think of leaving my palace. Without my prince, it became just a place.

Chapter 34
Auntie Belle

"No act of kindness, no matter how small,
is ever wasted." - Aesop.

MY CHILDREN AND GRANDCHILDREN were a great source of comfort to me after my husband Patrick's passing. They made it that I could begin a new life. They were there to listen to me, advise me and most importantly to show me that I mattered to them.

Even though three of my kids had moved out of Montreal, Susan to Toronto and the boys to Vancouver, they still made efforts to include me in their life by peppering the next few months and years with trips to see them.

In the spring of 2001, my sons bought me a ticket to Vancouver for a month. I was treated like a queen during that visit.

We wandered through the national parks with the trees reaching up almost to the clouds. We talked and laughed, and for a moment, I felt like I was a young mommy again. During the days they worked, I explored. I even hopped on a bus and found myself on a beach with the sun kissing my skin.

When I got back to Montreal, I sold the trailer home, and Jo-Ann helped me apply for low-income housing. The government agent who handled my application let me know it would take a while before I could get a spot and advised me to find an apartment in the meantime.

I wanted to stay in Chambly, and Carol helped me find a one-bedroom basement apartment. Once I had moved in, I began introducing myself to my neighbours. Some of them became friends. But of course, when you start getting to know your neighbours, you also get to know when something isn't quite right in their home. One of my new neighbours had a son. He would always smile and say hello when I would enter the complex. One evening, as I was coming home, he was sitting outside in the dark. It was cold, and I asked him why he wasn't in his apartment. He told me that he was not allowed to wake his mom after school. She was napping before work. I asked him if he was cold, and he said, "Yes." His name was Nick, and I introduced myself as Auntie Belle. It didn't take much coaxing to get him to come in and have hot soup, milk and cookies. The next morning his mother Tina knocked on my door. I invited her in for coffee.

We had often spoken since I had moved in, but never in-depth about our lives. Over coffee that morning, we got to know more about one another. Tina confided to me that she was an exotic dancer. I warned her to be careful of the monsters of the night. She confessed she would leave Nick home alone when she went off to work. Nick was only seven.

I asked Tina if she minded if Nick slept on my couch instead of being home alone and she could pick him up after her shift. She looked at me gratefully and said yes.

My family did not like this, "Mom if anything happens, she will accuse you." I paid them no mind. Helping them was the right thing to do. Nick would even stop by on the nights I wasn't watching him; to get some cookies and milk and say a quick hello. It felt so good to be useful again. My life had become much more comfortable over the years, I didn't worry about food or rent, but I hadn't changed who I was and what I believed; you don't judge others, you help and share.

I won't lie and say I loved living in my basement apartment; it was still a basement apartment. My experiences had made it that just the idea of living in a basement was not the best, but it was in a clean and new building and had one very attractive part to it; Baby Lorraine's house was up the street, and both Carol and Jo-Ann lived nearby.

I loved being closer to my girls and spending time with their families. I would walk down to Carol's house. She had a pool, and my daughters and their kids would gather over there to swim and spend time together. Other days we'd end up at Baby Lorraine's for a barbecue, once again the family together.

One summer day, I was over at Baby Lorraine's, and as usual, she refused to let me cook. I was sitting at the kitchen table just reading the weekly flyers when she went out to start the barbecue. A few minutes later, she flew into the house with her spatula in hand, screaming, "MOM, MOM."

"What's the problem?" I asked.

"MOMMY, there's a mouse in the barbecue!" Her eyes were as big as saucers.

"Give me that spatula," I said and marched out to the barbecue with Baby Lorraine trailing behind me a few steps back, scared to death. I opened the barbecue lid and wacked that mouse with the spatula and tossed the spatula back to her and said, "For fuck sakes, what's wrong with you? It's just a mouse! Thank God you were too young to remember the rats."

Baby Lorraine just stood there with her mouth open as I went back to reading my flyers. I was happy that the years of whack-a-rat or spraying the bugs hadn't marked her. They weren't the memories I wanted her to keep of her childhood.

All my kids had pushed past the difficulties in their childhoods. And more than just overcoming them, they had grown to be incredibly kind and generous grown-ups. They surrounded me with love. I must have done something right.

Darrell and Baby Lorraine had made a habit of renting a country cottage on the weekends, and they would invite me to go with them. Summer weekends filled with campfires, fireflies, and family became a staple in my life.

As fall came and the summer cottage weekends ended, I had the chance to make a few memories of my own with Carol, my daughter I had neglected in the past. With some of the money I had saved from the sale of the trailer I took a trip to Cuba with Carol, Lori and her kids. I loved sitting on the beach with the water touching the soles of my feet. One by one, it washed the grains of sand away, and one by one, I could feel a release; the hardships and losses receded into the ocean.

I feel like that trip cleansed me and turned the page forward. I never lost any of the love I felt for the men I lost. Each of them is still in my heart, but if I had concentrated on their physical loss, I would have been no more. My children and their love kept me in the mix, and I survived and found a way to thrive.

Chapter 35
In Memory Of Susan Ann Lessard

"When you are sorrowful look again in your heart, and you shall see that in truth you are weeping for that which has been your delight." - K.G.

IT TOOK MORE THAN seven years to get my place in low-income housing. By then, I had almost exhausted all of my savings.

Luckily Chambly had also introduced a free local bus, which allowed me to keep my independence and the few pennies I had left.

My low-income apartment was a short bus ride away from Baby Lorraine and Jo-Ann's, a ride I'd often take. On the days they were busy, I'd head to the grounds of Fort Chambly, and I'd stroll the day away, enjoying the kiss of sunshine on my face.

I didn't have too many responsibilities or chores to do, leaving me often at loose ends and I would try to find ways to keep busy. I would go to functions at the legion. I loved to help in the kitchen when they had dances. I could make finger sandwiches, you know! Finally, one place that welcomed my help in the kitchen.

But of course, there weren't dances every day and the days and weeks soon started to blend. I was nearing 80, and I guess it's to be expected that my life would have to slow down and that sometimes my mind would feel foggy. I'd call my kids, but I was confused as to why I had called them. Old age was setting in, and it was frustrating. I tried to ignore it the best I could.

By 2014, I wasn't as confident as I used to be setting off on a bus. Before, I had loved it when my kids would ask me to visit, but now I began making excuses not to go.

Going alone had become an ordeal. I had started forgetting little things, and my hearing and eyesight had worsened. I had missed my bus stops a few times because I hadn't realized where I was. I preferred staying near my apartment or taking a taxi. Inside my apartment, I felt safe, mostly. I had forgotten a meal or two on the stove. My mind had just wandered away from cooking, and the pan had burned to a crisp. It wasn't a big deal, but I did stop heating my food. I knew better than to admit that to the kids, though; they already thought so poorly of my cooking skills. Imagine if they knew that I had made such a mess. At night, from my balcony, I could hear the rush of water from the Richelieu River, and the sound would lull me with its soothing melody. I'd forget about my age, my aches and pains.

Susan tried to get me to visit her in Toronto. I kept cancelling at the last minute. She wasn't happy with me, and it was hard to explain to her that I wasn't feeling like myself, and I wasn't secure enough to go alone. All I could think of was what would happen if I forgot to get off the train? Just the idea scared me.

In October, I received another call from Susan, and she wanted to talk to me. This time it wasn't about visiting her, but I couldn't understand what she was saying. She spoke softly, and it seemed to be important, but I couldn't focus on her words.

Around December, my kids began calling me and telling me that "Susan is not well. We have to go see her." They would be bringing me, and I wouldn't be alone, so I agreed, and we went. Baby Lorraine, Darrell, Jo-Ann and Stephen. Everyone was quiet on the drive, but I was happy to have them all together. When we got to her hospital room, Susan was in bed, sitting cross-legged. I smiled and went to her, and she declared, "I have cancer, and I am going to die." This little five foot nothing mini- boss just threw it out there. "Die," I didn't understand why she said it. Why would she think that?

I kept looking into her eyes and face; she looked so sad it made me sad. I knew she was sick, but the rest made no sense to me. It was too much. I felt flustered. Baby Lorraine was telling Susan, "No, not now. We can fix this."

What did my Susan have? Why was everyone so worried? Susan was my healthy child, my mini-boss. She can't die. They kept talking, but their voices felt like they were far away. I could not focus. We hugged, and then we all left and went back to the car and headed home to Montreal. I knew Susan needed me; I just couldn't remember why. I hated how old age was affecting me. It would come back to me, is what I told myself and shrugged it off.

December 17, 2014, Darrell and Lorraine came to get me and drove me back to the Toronto hospital. I felt clear that day and knew it was bad. We arrived, and my Susan was asleep. They said she was in a medically induced coma.

Susan was pronounced dead from lung cancer 15 minutes later.

There is no greater pain than the loss of a child. I would never walk this earth whole again. She took a part of my heart with her. I will never be Belle, a mother of six again. I am supposed to be the one to be buried first, not my child.

This is not how this is supposed to happen. I am supposed to go before her. "God, no! She is my baby."

She was my strength, my guidance, my first-born. Susan lived the worst life of my six children; she sacrificed her childhood to help her siblings and me. Many nights she lay hungry, and still, she never complained. She never asked for anything.

I cried and cried, as did everyone in the room. We all felt this heavy loss with no understanding of why Susan had to leave us.

The day left me drained. My mind felt un-right, I felt unhinged, but I knew that it must be from the grief.

The next week went by with me in a daze. I don't know if I ate or who was around. I did know my boys wouldn't be at the funeral as René Baby-La-La had had surgery on his heart in Vancouver. Baby Lorraine kept explaining that to me. I let my daughters take charge of everything, and I just let my mind wander.

Where do I go from here? I have buried the three men I truly loved, I have just buried my daughter, and no parent should have to do this.

I dream many nights of Susan; she comes to me on a breeze, or a thought, or a whisper. When I close my eyes, I see her little face, that tiny little face, and feel the touch of her small hand in mine.

I have dedicated my life to my children, and I have loved and cared for my grandchildren and great-grandchildren. I sometimes ask and watch from my window for a surprise visit; it does not happen. I feel like screaming, "This is the time I need your help!" My kids say they have spoken to me already when I call, trying to reach out to them. I don't know if it is true. My mind isn't quite right.

Now with my fractured thoughts, I forget who has passed; maybe it's God's way of being merciful and making me blissfully unaware of my losses even though there are days I also remember them quite lucidly. But my fractured thoughts don't only affect the bad memories; they affect the simple happy things like my grandbabies' names. One thought remains clear; I don't want to be alone again.

Alzheimer's

"Today I bent the truth to be kind,
and I have no regret for I am far surer of
what is kind than I am of what is true."
- Robert Brault.

"I don't remember what she said,"

"What who said, Mommy?" Jo-Ann answered.

"What was my Doctor talking about?" Belle asked.

"Mommy, you have Alzheimer's."

"No, I don't. I am just getting old!"

After all the trials and years of struggle, Belle suffers her greatest loss of all, the loss of herself. Alzheimer's is robbing her of all she has known and all that she has; memories, spirit, and dignity.

We, her children, are having to say goodbye to our mother as she slips slowly away from us, and she is still here. It breaks our hearts.

I, Lorraine, will narrate what it's like to be with her through this. Jo-Ann and I have taken on the honour of caring for her as Alzheimer's ravages her mind.

Chapter 36
I Told You I'm Not Crazy

"I have been through a lot, and still a lot, never any peace for me." – Belle, 2020

ALONG WITH MOM AND most of my siblings, I also first thought she was just getting old. It was Jo-Ann who noticed little things like that she was repeating herself or forgetting well, forgetting pretty much everything! She would call us numerous times on the same day, forgetting we had just spoken.

It had begun after Patrick's passing and got worse after Susan left us. Mom seemed to understand that Susan wasn't with us any longer, but at the same time, she did not. I disregarded this obvious red flag, refusing to see it for what it was. Mom had undergone a blow after losing her husband and had now suffered the heart-wrenching pain of Susan's death. I felt it was normal for her to feel confused after so much loss.

I was not making light of her confusion, but I was making excuses for it. We were all dealing with heavy grief; who was I to fault her? I tried to see her more often because I thought it was also due to her being lonely. She had begun going by the Local Community Service Centre (CLSC) regularly, for aches and pains but mostly to talk with someone.

After a while, the CLSC banned her because she would make a fuss when they'd refuse to give her a consultation. I got frustrated with her when she would tell me about it—telling her to stop bugging them. I didn't understand the severity of her cry for help, which is what these visits to the CLSC were.

The CLSC staff contacted her doctor, who asked us to come in for a meeting about our mother. It was Jo-Ann who went.

She was the one that was with Mom the most during this period; she was also the one who felt there was something seriously wrong with Mom. Jo-Ann didn't confide in me her worries about our mother and the potential reason for the meeting. To be fair, I don't know if I would have believed her if she had.

The doctor requested that Mom be tested for Alzheimer's. Jo-Ann had prepared herself for this and asked many questions: how will it progress? Will it take time? Will it be fast? Will she be bedridden? The doctor explained how a counsellor from the CLSC had been assigned not only to Mom but to our whole family to help us walk through it.

When Jo-Ann called me, I was dumbfounded. It was like I had a curtain over my eyes; I knew something was awry with Mom but didn't really comprehend the depth of the problem until the curtain came up, and I had no choice but to see.

There was no shielding myself from the truth. I had to accept that everything might not be alright. Now began the long wait to find out if Mom had this terrible disease.

We would take Mom to many diagnostic tests over the next eight months. Each time she would say to us, "You know I am not crazy. I just forget." Jo-Ann started to leave notes on her fridge because she couldn't remember her appointments anymore.

I had to learn how to deal with her and not be angry with her. It was hard when I'd be confronted with situations that didn't make sense. Mom had begun to lose a lot of weight on her already slender frame. Jo-Ann and I found out Mom was not eating. She tried to hide it and tell us that she was, but it was plain to see she wasn't. We would go to her apartment and throw out food that had gone bad because Mom hadn't cooked it for fear of leaving the stove on. Frustrated, we tried to buy her prepackaged frozen meals, where all she would have to do is microwave them. For a while, it worked, then Mom seemed to forget to eat them. We tried a food service that would bring her meals. She complained that the main meal didn't taste good and would leave it in her fridge. For someone who had sent us to school with sardine and mustard sandwiches, we couldn't believe how picky she had gotten. The only thing she ate was the dessert out of the meal. Mom had never had a sweet tooth. She was a lover of chips and everything salty, so it caught us by surprise that she'd always finish the dessert. The CLSC counsellor explained how people with Alzheimer's taste buds begin to drop, and the only thing that remains high is a craving for sweets. It was exasperating. Every way we'd try to fix things, she would refuse, and we would fail.

I was still working full-time, and Jo-Ann, although she tried to be there as much as possible, it was never enough to prevent all the small yet significant issues that came up.

Mom began to have little panic episodes, worried that she would mess up simple tasks like pushing her pin code for purchases, she would ask the cashiers to do it. Soon she shared her pin code with anyone who came in contact with her. By doing so, some people took advantage of her and depleted her meagre savings. Jo-Ann had to go and deal with Mom's bank, shocked they hadn't noticed or sent word to her family that unusual activity was going on in her account.

Finally, all the medical test results were in; we were called to come in with her to the doctor's office. This time I went with them. Mom was anxious about her results. Her doctor confirmed what we feared: Mom had Alzheimer's. Her doctor explained to us what the disease meant. I had to leave the room many times; I was overwhelmed and didn't want my mother to see me cry. Mom listened to the doctor, nodded and said, "Yes, I understand but I need some time to process my feelings." She then turned to us and told us, "I am not crazy. I told you, I have Alzheimer's."

It wasn't long until everyone in her low-income building knew she had been diagnosed with Alzheimer's. The residents started to take advantage of her inability to make good decisions and preyed on her. They began to take many of her things when we were not there, and some precious keepsakes: Dad's wedding ring and military pins. Then she started to give everything away because she didn't know better, even her furniture. I always remember my mom saying, "A poor person doesn't call another poor person poor. They give it to the other person."

Unfortunately, this was not a case of Mom giving out of generosity. She did not know why she was giving. When we were going through some of her things and found so much missing, we would become so frustrated. "Mom, where is this, and where is that?" Mom would shrug her shoulders and slouch down and hang her head just like a child. "I don't know," she would say in a little voice reminiscent of a child who just got caught taking cookies out of the cookie jar. Defeated, we would throw our hands up. There was no way for us to stop it or find out who had taken the items. We knew something had to change.

Jo-Ann seemed to be able to deal better with it than I. Jo-Ann found a quiet fortitude. I, however, did not, at that time. Mom has been my strength all my life. I depended on her always being there because she had taught me how to become who I was. I know it sounds selfish, but it was hard for me to accept that Mom could no longer be my pillar of strength. I did not want to accept it, but I knew I must. It was my turn to hold her up.

I thanked God that I had Jo-Ann to help me.

Jo-Ann and I began asking each other these questions. "What are we going to do? Which one of us can take care of her?" "She is going to get worse. Do you have the ability to help her through this until the end?" "Do you know what to do?"

The only thing we knew for sure was that her low-income seniors' apartment was no longer an option for her. Mom, Belle, needed a safe place where her kindness and her illness would not be exploited.

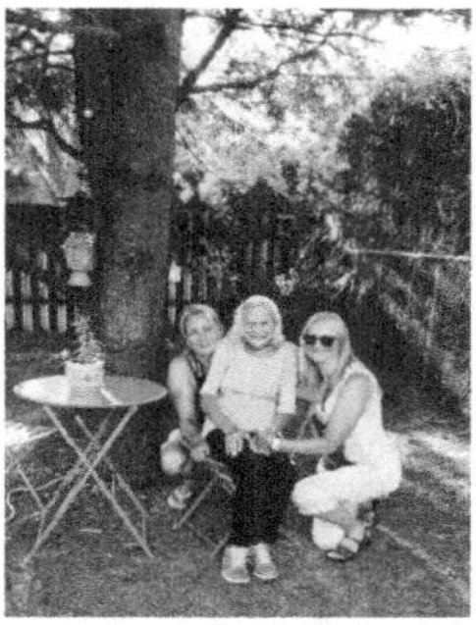

Chapter 37
A Safe Place

"I am not leaving yet, I talked to my friend, God, and he said I can stay, it's not time yet." – Belle, 2019

THE CLSC GAVE US a list of reputable senior homes. Jo-Ann visited them with a friend who had been through this with her parents.

We settled on one across the river, a 10-minute drive away from both our homes. We chose it not only because of the location but also because of the services offered. There were standard emergency pull cords next to the bed and in the bathroom. The home also provided a full-time nurse, laundry service and all meals. The only catch was that we had to convince Mom to go.

"Mommy, we have to start packing," I said.

"Why? I don't have to move." "Yes, Mom, you do. You can't stay here on your own anymore. We found you a nice apartment not far from here."

"I won't be put in a hospital!" She answered back.

Being put in a hospital seemed to be her biggest fear. We had this same conversation repeatedly as we tried to get her ready for the move. She would forget it each time.

By moving day, things had gotten out of hand in her apartment. We arrived, and many pieces of furniture were missing. "Where did the table go, Mommy?"

Mom slumped down and answered in a childlike voice, "I don't know."

It felt like if we didn't hustle and get her out of there, there would be nothing left to move. Carol, Jo-Ann and I worked together to pack up all her belongings. It was a sad day; Mom watched us load up the truck and was lost as to what to do to help. It took us a few trips to bring all her things to the residence. Mom stayed in her apartment until the last piece of furniture had been put in the truck.

After it had been loaded up, she came with us to the seniors' care residence, her new home. Her home was on the terrace level in a spacious room with a separate bathroom and patio doors opening up to a little deck on the grass.

Mom helped us put some things away. Carol and Jo-Ann had already set up a lot of her belongings before Mom had come in. We had thought that if she walked into a room where all her things were set up, she would feel more comfortable. We made sure to bring many of the items that she loved: a loveseat in the most beautiful fabric of cream with a sprinkling of peonies in pink, her bedspread that also had peonies in the print, a lovely antique white dresser and matching coffee table, and a nice electric fireplace, which also was the stand for her TV. Jo-Ann added some warm touches by putting all the family pictures on display. It creates a homey, cozy feeling as soon as you enter. The staff admired the room and remarked on how pretty it looked. Belle smiled and said, "My girls did it."

We felt proud to have provided Mom with a safe, beautiful place.

When it was time for us to leave, Mom turned to us and said, "Why did you bring all of my clothes here? I am not staying HERE!"

"Yes, Mom, this is your home now," I said.

She looked right into my eyes, so deep it felt like it reached my soul and found that place that only she could touch and then swiftly, she turned away from me.

"Mom, this is your place," Jo-Ann said. "We want you to be safe. It's not a prison. You can come and go as you please. You can still come over to our houses, and we will still take you out shopping and for breakfast."

The residence consisted of three sections. In the first section, called Maison 1, residents were allowed to go freely in and out of the building. In the second section, called Maison 2, residents were kept inside. Maison 3, the third section was for the residents who needed the heaviest care. Mom was in the first section and would be able to go out as much as she wanted.

It took a lot of persuading, but by evening she accepted that it was her home. We should have felt relieved, but when we closed the door to her new place, the look on her face was devastating to see. Jo-Ann and I got in the car, and we cried. We cried because our lives had changed forever. Every day we were losing a little of our mother. Every day she was losing a bit of her life as a strong woman, Belle.

She had always been the one who took care of everyone, and now Mom had to depend on others. She fought it the only way she knew how; she cleaned. Mom started to wash her clothes in the bathtub and refused to let the cleaning staff tidy up her place. We would visit, and all her laundry would be hanging off of everything.

"I know how to clean my house," she would argue. Eventually, the cleaning staff would come and clean her room when she was out for lunch. Even they didn't want the wrath or trouble of dealing with our Tuffy Mom. Although she had a hard time letting others help her, she was still Mom: friendly, talkative and outgoing. She quickly became the social butterfly of the place.

She would commute through all the connected buildings and spread her smiley face around, stopping to say hi and chat with patients and staff alike.

Mom often tells the story of how she laid down the rules at the seniors' home, and she tells it like this: "When Darrell came by to visit with Baby Lorraine, I took him on a tour. As we passed the other residents and staff, I introduced him as my bodyguard and told them they better be nice to me or else. Darrell chuckled when I said it, but I stayed serious. I know the stories of abuse or neglect. Not going to happen to this old lady! Tuffy Belle still has some tricks."

But these highly funny moments were often followed by lows. There were not enough activities in the residence to keep our active mother busy. She would often call us crying on the phone, "Why have you put me here? I never abandoned you, children? Why? I always put you first. How could you leave me?"

Mom asked to be seen by a psychologist. Mom never used the word psychologist; she used the words "a doctor to talk to." From her previous bout with depression, she understood that she couldn't wait to have a breakdown. She needed help. She had asked her councillor from the CLSC to set it up for her. That was one of the moments when she demonstrated such a lucid train of thought that it felt like Mom wasn't dealing with this awful Alzheimer's illness. There were many moments of lucidity, and Mom maintained her way of life as much as she could. She had always been independent, walking, taking a bus or a taxi to get around. She continued to do it, not waiting to be taken out by us.

Although the home allowed the residents in Mom's section to go out by themselves, they still kept tabs on them. Often I would get a phone call. "Your mother is taking the bus by herself."

I would tell them it was okay because I wanted it to be. I wanted her to be normal, just to be Mom again. I have spent these years as her cheerleader. It was silly, but Belle was my Hero, and she had to do everything she used to do because, selfishly, I wanted her to. I could not accept her being someone different. Then Mom started talking about going for a walk by herself by the water. "No, Mom, you can't do that." Isabella Pearl Lawrence cannot swim, and even if she could, the rapids would sweep her away. The residence was just up the street from the rapidly flowing Richelieu River. Mom did not take the news well and spent some time sulking and trying to sneak off. She loved her freedom to come and go. Telling her she could not have this independence broke her heart, and she started to blame us for her dependence on everyone. I don't know how many times we pleaded with her not to go out without us.

"I will not go, I promise," she would say. Unfortunately, this was not true, and more extreme measures had to be taken. We would need to move her to a new room in the second section of the residence with full lockdown and coded entry.

She didn't take well to the restrictions. She lashed out, and her words hurt us, but this was not about us. It was about our Mom, Belle, who was now a desperate soul attacked by the mercilessness of Alzheimer's. We adjusted to hearing things that tore at our hearts, telling ourselves this wasn't Mom's words; this was the illness. Someone told me, at the beginning, it is her family that will feel the pain of the disease, and I thought that is a selfish way of looking at things. Now I know what they mean.

Chapter 38
My Eyes Are Opened

"If I was no longer here, then I won't be alone any longer." – Belle, 2019

EVERY TIME WE WOULD go to visit Mom, we would ready ourselves to be met with a new surprise. It's almost like, "What's behind door number three? A new Mom? A new adventure?"

Some days Jo-Ann and I would arrive, and Mom would be wearing maybe three shirts or four pairs of socks, and it was 90 degrees outside. Mom would get frustrated or outright refuse when we would tell her that she had to remove the extra clothing. Her reaction would be that of a tired child when you're trying to dress them for winter. They stiffen up and act up as if to say, "No way are you putting it on or taking it off."

Mom was slim, but her strength was extraordinary. "NO," she would declare, "I don't want to change my clothes." I figured out a way to deal with these situations. I would hold her close, hum and dance. Mom would try to wiggle out and push against me, but I was stronger than her and wouldn't allow her to move away.

She would start to laugh, and her thoughts would change from angry ones to happy ones. After dancing, she would let us dress her. It worked every time.

Jo-Ann had a more challenging time dealing with Mom's new bouts of lack of common sense. Jo-Ann is incredibly logical and was accustomed to Mom being a no-nonsense type of person. She had understood in the beginning when Mom was forgetful, but now it was a new ballgame. Mom was irrational and would often not listen. I would tell Jo-Ann to find humour in the silly things she said, think of it as the odd stuff toddlers do or say. We can't get upset; we have to figure out ways to change her thoughts. I would shift the conversation if it was going nowhere or when I could see Mom was getting herself riled up. I would say or write something silly on the whiteboard that I carried due to Mom's hearing loss. Mom would laugh, and her mind would move on from her original odd or disturbing thought.

A new irrational idea crept up in our mother's mind and stayed unexpectedly for a few months. Mom, who loved men, was attracted to a resident and he to her. They wanted to get married. We met him, and he seemed to be a nice guy, but the whole scheme was preposterous. "No!" said Jo-Ann, firmly. "No. You can hang out together, but no marriage." He didn't have Alzheimer's, and we were worried he was scamming her. Mom's hearing was almost gone, and her Alzheimer's was progressing; why would he want to marry her when they could hardly communicate or hold a conversation? She persisted with the idea for a while, but our worry and angst were for naught. After half a year, Mom did not even remember him. She knew she had seen him before but had already forgotten his name. Alzheimer's waits for no one; it takes away a memory one stem at a time. When someone would meet Mom for the first time, they couldn't tell how badly the disease affected her. She was friendly and outgoing, and that, combined with her physical appearance, still attracted people. She was quite beautiful when she was dressed up, and her ability to walk compared to the many incapacitated residents gave her an air of being healthy. Looks were deceiving. Her healthy appearance also seemed to confuse the staff at the residence. They believed she could do much more than she was able to. Mom needs to be assisted and watched for all her basic care activities.

Mom had stopped washing herself in her delicate areas and had also gotten into the habit of hiding her toilet paper (thinking someone would steal it). The missing toilet paper made it so that she wasn't wiping herself after using the washroom on top of not washing daily. The staff, seeing our happy-go-lucky mother, must have thought she was capable of handling her basic care. Neither Jo-Ann nor I knew about her not washing. We took it for granted that she was thoroughly looked after. That assumption had heavy repercussions.

One morning as we opened her door, we were met by a very distressing sight. Mom was sitting listlessly on the bed and told us, "I don't feel good." Her arms were dangling, she was crouched down and her voice was weak. I was terrified, I thought that something in her was shutting down and her life was in danger. Immediately I went to get the nurse. She came right away to my mother's room. Her blood pressure was taken. It was high and she was worried. She called an ambulance. I was nervous, pacing in her room, my hands shaking. Jo-Ann got Mom dressed as we waited for what seemed like an eternity for the ambulance to get there.

As soon as the paramedics loaded her into the ambulance, Jo-Ann and I rushed to the hospital.

She had a major urine infection that the residence nurse hadn't noticed. The hospital informed us of the dire circumstances if she was not treated right away. They also weighed her. Mom weighed a meagre 85 pounds. The hospital was concerned. They decided to keep her until she put the weight back on, mixing her soups with weight gain powder and adding an Ensure supplement to drink with every meal. The staff at the residence hadn't been watching to see if she was eating her meals. I was shocked when the hospital's doctor told me her weight. How had I let this happen? I knew she was slim, but not that her weight had dropped so much. I felt like I had neglected her care.

I only fully understood how thin she was once I bathed her at the hospital. She was not bruised or scarred but seeing the bones with just skin hanging off of her, I turned and splashed water on my face. I didn't want her to see me crying.

She looked so frail, weak and small. In my eyes, Mom was an Amazonian warrior; strong, fit and larger than life. What had happened? Mom was as tall as I am when she was younger. But in the shower, I towered over her. For a long time, I had just thought Mom was dealing with a mental disease, but now I had to open my eyes to the physical parts of Mom's plight. She had arthritis in her neck, making it so that she couldn't lift her head and had a tendency to cast her eyes downward. And she had a large lump on the top of her back that doesn't allow her to stand straight anymore.

The fragility of who Mom had become and how important she was to me was brought home that day. Jo-Ann and I went by daily while she was at the hospital. Providing her care, ensuring Mom ate her meals and that she washed properly. We resolved to continue the habit when she returned to the residence. It took a toll on us. The CLSC offered us a spa day, donated to the family of Alzheimer's patients. Jo-Ann and I didn't take them up on it. It was a kind gesture, wanting to provide us with a break, but we couldn't accept. We felt an overwhelming feeling of guilt every time we spent a day away from her or did something fun without her. Even on shopping trips to home decor shops, we'd feel bad for not bringing her. Thoughts of, "Oh, Mom would like that, she should be here," were constant. Our hearts were also heavy with regret for having missed the signs of Mom's deteriorating health, and we couldn't allow ourselves to miss even one more precious moment with her. Mom's counsellor from the CLSC kept telling us, "She doesn't have a sense of time; she won't know if you are not here for one day."

We would reply, "Yes, but we would know."

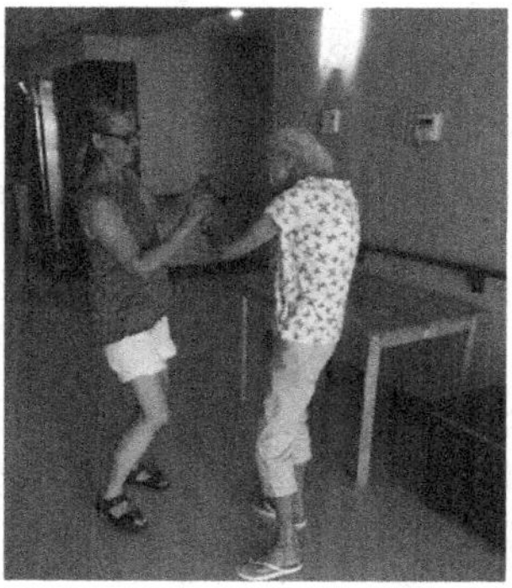

Conclusion
I Am Belle, You Are?

"When we dance, can we do it again?" – Belle, 2020

EVEN THOUGH JO-ANN AND I were there almost every day, Mom would see us and ask, "Where have you been?" She would forget we were just there. Then one day, the question changed as she looked at me. "Who are you? What's your name?" I smiled, hugged her and scribbled on the whiteboard, "Lorraine."

She said, "Really?"

She didn't know who I was. I went home and cried like a baby. I told myself that I would have to accept the eventual loss of my Mom while she is still on this Earth. And guess what? I still haven't. That day stays engraved in my mind; it was the first time in my life that my mom did not know me. Darrell held me and told me that night, "Lorraine, your mom didn't forget you. She forgot your name, but when you kiss and hug her, she will know who you are. It will be your scent, your touch when you embrace, and your chi. It will trigger an emotion attached between you two that even God can't end."

I hold on to those words from Darrell like a lifeline each time she asks me, "Really, you are my baby?" or "Lorraine, who gave you that name?"

I can't describe my feelings well. I have faith that she will never forget her baby in her deepest heart of hearts, but it's hard when confronted by her memory lapses towards me.

There are days when I find her funny when her face fills with astonishment when I tell her I'm hers. She looks so surprised, and I feel an overwhelming amount of love and loss. I miss her every day.

Mom is mostly deaf now. She doesn't hear us unless we scream in her ear, something I mostly refuse to do. Her thoughts are scrambled, and there are bad days when she can't string more than two words together, and some days nothing at all.

Mom doesn't remember taking off her clothes at night or putting them on in the morning. Brushing her teeth, combing her hair, cleaning herself, simple things we take for granted are all gone from her thoughts.

Her spirit remains, and for that, I am thankful. On the good days, we have fun together.

Mom still has that little devil in her.

She makes us laugh, makes us cry, and gives us the best hugs ever.

When we are out in nature, we see the Belle of before; our mother shines through.

We take long walks along the Richelieu River, and her face lights up with joy. Mom becomes animated and rambles on about the trees and how they are giants just waiting for someone to need their shelter, and she turns towards the river to smell the air blowing off it and says, "This is beautiful." She stops to pet the cats that always seem to find her on our walks, and if mothers with their babies pass us along the way, she tells them, "I love you."

We stroll inside the residence when the weather doesn't allow us to take her out. Mom has that same enthusiasm that she has when she sees the families outside and when she sees the staff when they pass us in the halls; Mom grabs their hand and says, "I love you."

Mom is now happy in Maison 2. We decorated her room the same as we had done in Maison 1. When we took her over to see it, she cried, "You did this for me?" Yes, we nodded. It pleased us to see her marvel at her new yet old things.

But before her move into Maison 2, Mom had to temporarily stay in Maison 3. Jo-Ann and I thought it to be the saddest place we had ever seen. The residents there are like lost souls left to die. Every day they go through the same routine; needles, medications, and food. After the food, they sit or sleep in chairs in the common room, urinate, and wait for their diapers to be changed. Jo-Ann and I would dread walking into Maison 3.

Even Mom noticed how depressing this section was. During one of our visits, she blurted out, "I'm not as bad as these guys! I don't belong here!" We burst out laughing. She was right; she didn't belong there.

The staff works hard in Maison 3, trying to provide all of the residents' basic care needs, but they require more than basic care. They need human touch, kindness and smiles. They mostly require interaction.

One day, as we were taking my mom out for a stroll, she stopped in the middle of the common room. The staff had music playing from a CD player, and I guess it was the music's vibration that caught her attention. She started to dance.

We watched her as she hummed and swayed to the rhythm. It wasn't long before some of the residents got out of their chairs and joined her. The ones who couldn't get up began to tap their feet and clap to the beat. My breath was taken away by the scene. I joined in, as did Jo-Ann, and we laughed and smiled and danced.

We spoke to her brother Doug about her joy of dancing and humming. He confided in us how they had danced with their mother Zita, every morning. We had always known Mom loved to dance but never knew why. Now it makes sense. Mom, Belle was holding tight to her happiness, to Zita. Belle will always get the last say. When she saw the trial cover of this book, her eyes lit up, and she smiled. She didn't stutter her words.

"That is Belle, that is me. We need to give this to the world."

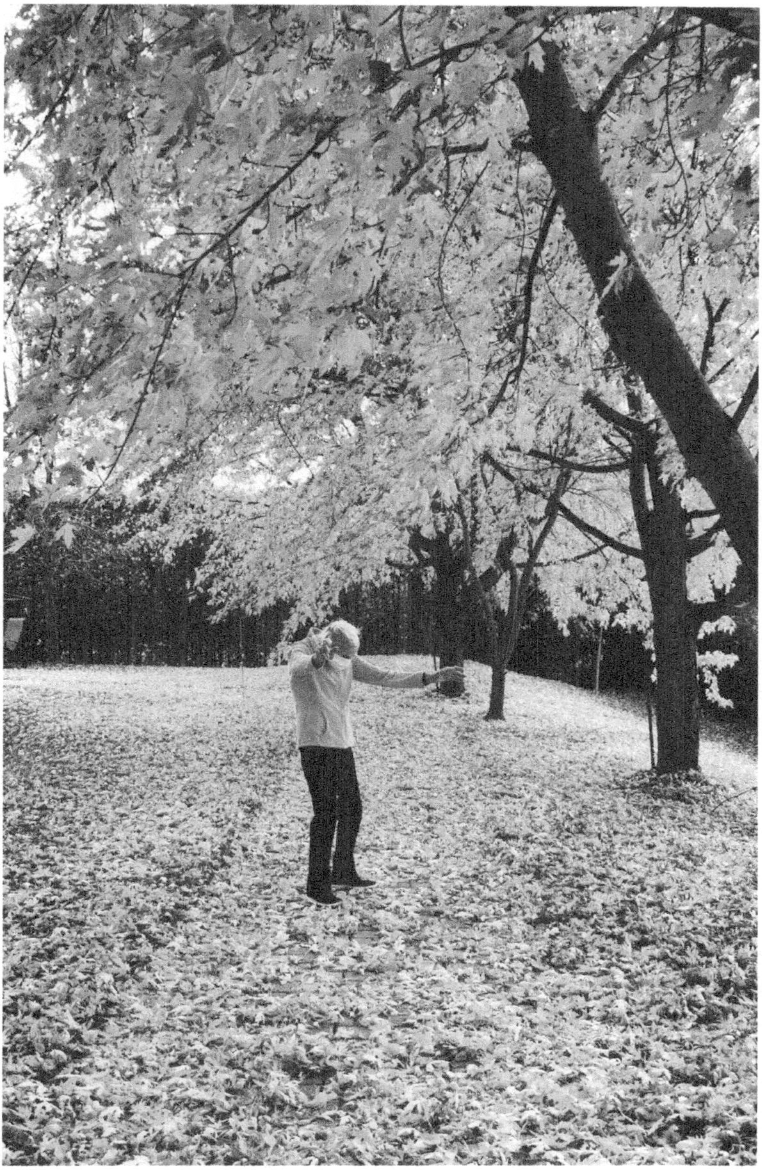

Belle, 2020

ACKNOWLEDGEMENTS

Darrell, my love, my husband, your encouragement and determination not to let me read you one little paragraph all through this tells me you want to embrace Dancing with Belle in its full beauty. Without you, Darrell and your encouragement, it might not have happened. You are my Hero.

Darrell Jr., and Kyell, my sons you are my greatest accomplishment. I know you are proud of me and I love you both.

Daniel, my big brother, was my source of a lot of dates and names and stories the way he remembered. Daniel, you had to revisit a past you left behind, and I thank you for your bravery in opening old wounds for me. I know it was not easy, but you did it!

Thank you. Without your encouragement and your eagerness for this book to be published, maybe it would never have happened.

Big Brother, my defender, Mom said you are your mother's son; you came from an angry little boy and a troubled young man into our Mother's Hero, you set the bar high for all of us. I love you, my Big Brother. You make our mom proud.

My little Mom Susan left us in the year 2014, but her stories never left my memories. You showed me how to love by loving me. As long as I live, you live, for you taught me, you fed me, took care of me. Although you are not of this Earth, you are forever a part of me.

Susan, I was listening when you were telling me everything. I only wanted to make you proud with this book, for pride and love is all you ever have shown me. Although you are not of this Earth, you are forever a part of me. Miss you, my little mom.

Jo-Ann, my sister, you have been there for Mom and me while you fight your own battle. I thank you for your stories.

Thank you to Uncle Doug for your way of setting the record straight and telling it like it was. Also, thank you for your service and bravery for our country. Your love of your sister is undying.

Thank you, Aunt Loy, for reaching into a part of your big sister that I know was sometimes painful for you. I realize some stories were too sad, and you didn't want me to know; The things no one should have to endure, especially your big sister some of it had to be left in that old trunk not to see the light of day again. This, I understand.

Evie Belaiv, for your French translations at all hours of the day, thank you, sweetie.

Before I thank the team at Smiling Eyes Press, I have to thank all of our friends out there, Oss for Ontario, Oss for Ottawa. I cannot thank all of you enough for all your support of this story and your support for me, your friend. Thank you, Sisters of the Wave. I love you all.

Thank you, *Smiling Eyes Press*. From a meeting over coffee in Timmy's, wow, what a journey. I thank you for making a dream of a lifetime for Belle come to life. I truly enjoyed the personal connection with Dounia; I have found a friend in you. I believe we knew each other before, maybe in another lifetime, for we just picked up where we left off. Thank you, my friend, Dounia.

Richard, you make my mom proud. Thank you for your dedication. You took my vision of her stories and wrapped it up in the most beautiful of bows. What a cover.

DEDICATION & TRIBUTES TO BELLE

"Belle would dance with our Mom Zita every day. Belle always took care of Loy and me. We always got along, we were friends, and I always loved Belle."

- *Douglas Lawrence*

"A few words about my beloved sister, Isabella Pearl Lawrence, called Belle. She was always a nice sister to me. She made sure I was safe and looked after. Doug and Belle dragged me along everywhere. How Belle managed to feed and house her kids was a miracle. No help from the city or charities at first, she babysat and cleaned houses, and she babysat for me also. Belle's first love was her kids. All children loved Belle. Belle was a bugger.

She was daring and had a hard head, and determined to be her own person. My sister was always sweet, like our mom. May we always love and respect her as she deserves. I could go on forever about Belle, a loving and vibrant woman. I hope you all know she was a wonderful proof of loving her family."

- *Loy Tombs*

"I think the hard part is also that I cannot call her because she cannot hear. All her life, she loved everyone. When she disciplined me, I never took it personally because I know I drove her nuts.

There are all types of ways we lose someone, but to lose your mind is a long, slow punishment for her family. Mom is what all moms should be. The six kids are all doing well in life because of her strength to never give up and not be afraid to protect. With mom's positive attitude, I do not ever feel bad about us having a tough time; she never showed weakness when we were around. Mom and Dad, no matter what, found a way to keep us together. Even as an adult, we all counted on her, and she never said no. It's sad kids grow up, leaving mom with no more responsibilities.

Every grandchild and great grandchild were and are loved and cared for as her own child. After all the hard and happy times we had with her, it's so sad the mind is going. Remember to never give up on her. There is always a good day every day as long as her feet touch the earth. I love her dearly with all my soul.

Mom, no one could be as great a mom as you are. I love and miss you all the time; when the world is not sick, I will come to see you. Your smile opens hearts. Sorry, I am not there, but I can see you in my mind and heart. I Love you.

This is a poem I believe most represents my mom:

"Mother is the essence of love, a constant source of patience and understanding. Her gentle touch, reassuring smile, and endless devotion are a source of strength through the years and across the miles. Mother is wisdom, guidance, and beauty, whose life experiences guide her children on the path to happiness." - Unknown author - Love you Mom."

- Daniel Lessard

"Unfortunately, I am having a really hard time speaking on Mom. I can't express my thoughts. It's so hard, Mom is here but not. It's a horrible illness; it takes my loved one from my soul."

- Rene Jr. Lessard

"I don't know why, but I struggled with writing something so much. Every time I tried, I would cry. I couldn't really find the words to say how I feel. I just can't deal with the pain and sadness of it all.

We are so blessed that we can show her our love every day. Even if the words escape me, I know she knows how much I love her. Alzheimer's can't take that away!"

- Jo-Ann Carter

"I have searched for the moments and cannot for the life of me remember a time when any harsh words ever graced my lips against this woman Isabella.

From the moment we met, I was her guardian Angel, and she became Mom No 2. Isabella welcomed me with open arms, and still today, they are stretched wide. Isabella always gave me a big hug and a kiss, always a little close to the mouth, haha. She has done this with all her children and grandchildren, and I would say, "Great Grandchildren," all the while waiting for the punchline, "Not on the mouth, Mother."

This is a special bond that has forever been cast. And through our lives, it has never been broken. She has been Mom and, for me, revered as such. She has been held in my heart with the greatest of love and respect. I have been a witness to her life and can testify she has been the heart of the glue that binds. For you, knowledge of love comes from selfless unmeasured and truly drawn upon in our times of need. Oh, how the sands of time cover what is too difficult to remember, yet she bears her strength even today when she is put aside for a more favourable ending. She will not go hidden, for her strength will not allow it. Isabella, Mom is still with you because you cannot change what has been done for you! For us."

- *Darrell Henegan*

"Did you ever watch the fireflies skim across the grass in the darkness of a warm summer night? Did you ever watch the butterflies flutter their wings in delight? Have they ever sat on your hand as gentle as summer rain? It feels magical yet comforting.

Mom makes me feel this way with those warm blue eyes and that sweet lined face that tells a tale of life, the twists and turns. I see love, a love so great it has made me see all the beauty in life.

Mom has shown me never to quit, and what we give comes back, so be good, share, love, and stand up every time you fall, no matter how often, and help anyone who needs it; it may be you someday.

Love is eternal, and when I see the beauty of a simple ripple in the water, the scent of the air by the river, the beauty of the twisting branches that have fought against the winds and rain and ice with nowhere to go but up and still offer shelter. Mom mimics the water and the trees as she has also sheltered us through life's struggles.

I will forever hear your song in my heart. When we dance, it's our dance, a private moment in time. Our story cannot possibly end here."

- Baby Lorraine

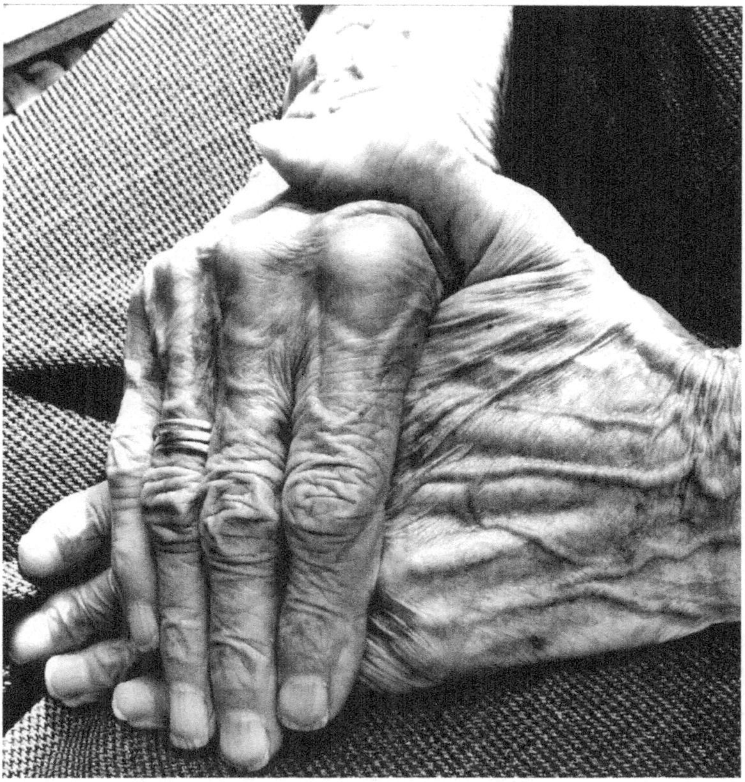

The hands are a reflection of our life, a record of the advantage or disadvantage we have lived. These are Belle's hands: many years of scrubbing other people's laundry on a washboard, cleaning of other people's homes, many hands held of her babies and the babies of others she cared for, and many smacks on the butt of her children and also held in prayer. If you hold them, they are as soft as a baby's bottom. They are as strong as the great Amazonian Queen Otrera yet as gentle as a breeze on the trees. Our Belle. Our Mom.

Alzheimer Society of Canada

www.alzheimer.ca

ABOUT THE AUTHOR

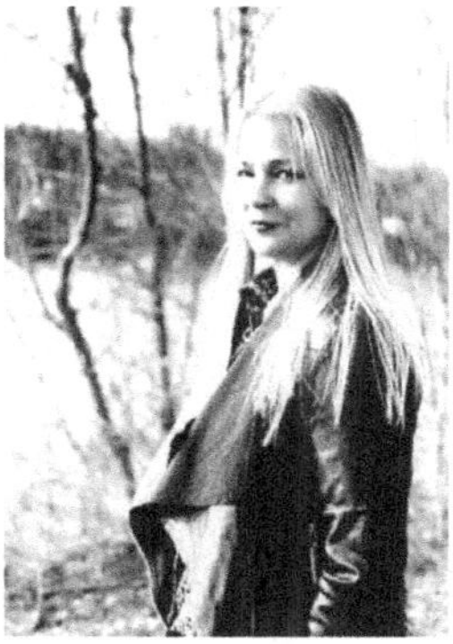

Lorraine was born in Montreal, Quebec, Canada, and is the youngest of six children. She is the author of Dancing with Belle, a tale of her mother's life and battle with Alzheimer's.

She lives on the South Shore with her husband Darrell and her unruly dog Thor. Lorraine is also the mother to two wonderful men, Darrell Jr. and Kyell, and grandmother to one perfect grandson, Little Lion. Dancing with Belle is her first but hopefully not last book.

AUTHOR'S NOTE

I have tried to be as accurate as possible telling the story of Isabella Pearl Lawrence. The dates and events depicted in this book are in no way meant to harm or embarrass anyone mentioned. This is the story as I know it, and I am responsible for my words. It is as accurate as I know it. It is Belle's story.

Other Books by Smiling Eyes Press

Stop the Denial: A Case for Embracing the Truth about Fitness, by Richard Tardif, June, 2017.

Still in Denial: Five Reasons for Embracing the Truth About Fitness, by Richard Tardif, April, 2019.

Your House Stinks: How to Survive Homeownership, by Ivan Mose, March, 2020.

Insider Secrets to INTERNET SAFETY: Advice From a Professional Hacker, by Terry Cutler, April, 2020.

The Joy of Life: Now What?
by Olga Munari, July, 2020.

My Side of the Kaniá:tara:
A Non-Indigenous Perspective on Reporting in Indigenous Communities, by Richard Tardif, May, 2020.

The Joy of Cancer: A Journey of Self-Discovery,
By Olga Munari and Kim Mecca, December, 2020.

Made in the USA
Monee, IL
04 November 2026

67379467R00154